ESSENTIALLY
HAPPY

ESSENTIALLY HAPPY

3 Simple Answers from Mother Nature
for Overcoming Depression

SPECIAL EDITION

REBECCA LINDER HINTZE, M.Sc.
with Stephanie Gunning

🅒 VISIUMGROUPLLC
Ashburn, Virginia

This book is intended as a reference volume only, not as a medical manual. The information given here is designed to help you make informed decisions about your health and well-being. It is not intended as a substitute for any treatment that may have been prescribed by your doctor. If you suspect that you have a medical problem, we urge you to seek competent medical help.

Mention of specific companies, organizations, or authorities in this book does not imply endorsement by the authors or publisher, nor does mention of specific companies, organizations, and authorities imply that they endorse this book, its authors, or the publisher.

Brief excerpts in this book written by Rebecca Linder Hintze have previously appeared in *Living Healthy & Happily Ever After* by Rebecca Linder Hintze and Dr. Susan Lawton, copyright © 2012; and in *Healing Your Family History* by Rebecca Linder Hintze, copyright © 2006.

Cover design by Quinn Curtis
Interior design by Gus Yoo
Author photo by Shane Hintze

Copyright © 2014 by Rebecca Linder Hintze. All rights reserved. No part of this book may be reproduced or transmitted in any form or by any means, electronic or mechanical, including photocopying, recording, or any other information storage and retrieval system, without the express written permission of the publisher. For permission, email: info@essentiallyhappy.com.

Ordering information: Special discounts are available on quantity purchases by corporations, associations, and others. For details, contact orders@essentiallyhappy.com.

978-0-9724297-2-6 (special edition)
978-0-9724297-3-3 (paperback)
978-0-9724297-4-0 (ebook)

To Shane

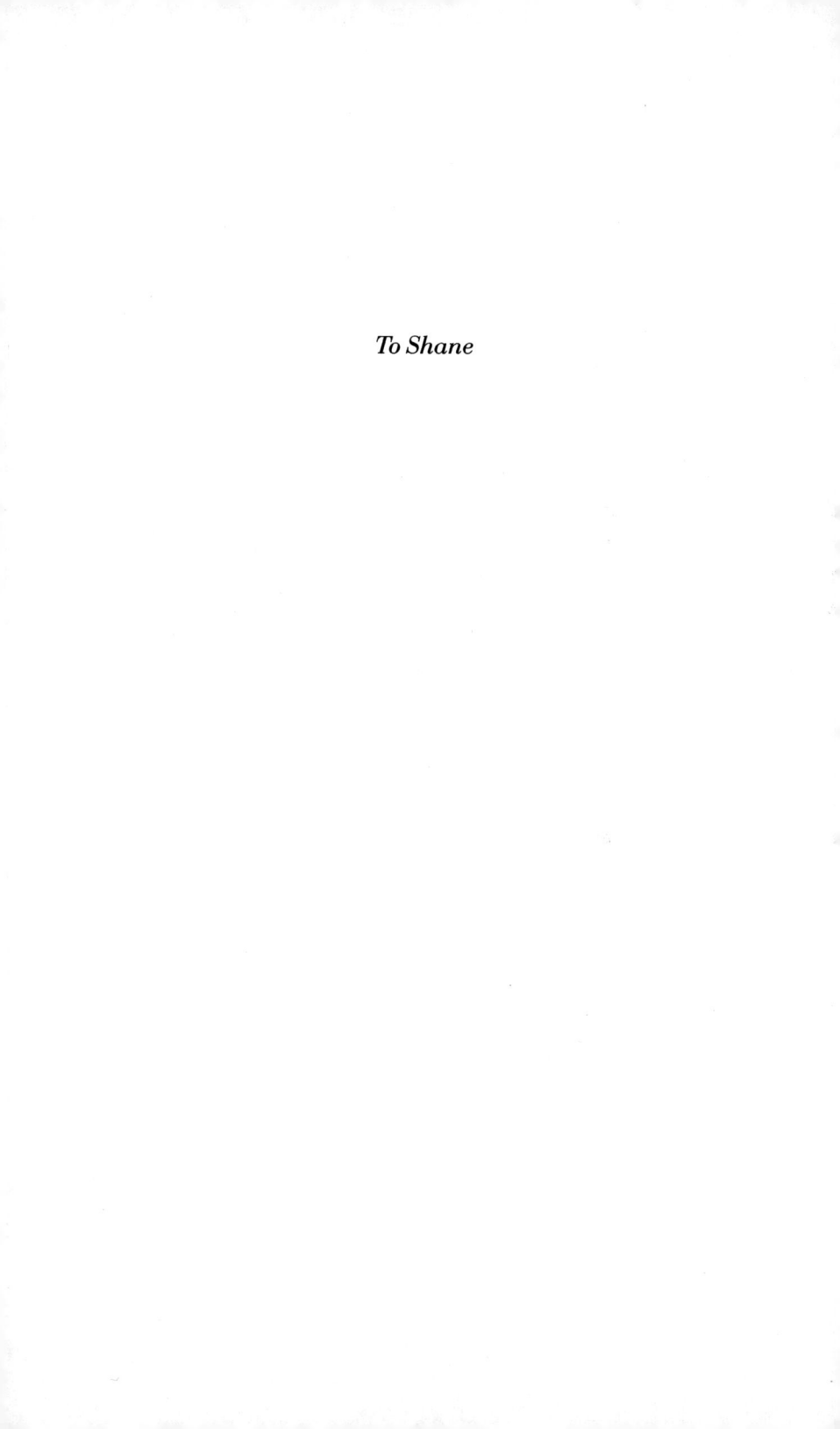

Contents

Introduction: Overcoming Depression Naturally 1

Mother Nature's Answer 1: Happy Nutrition 9

Mother Nature's Answer 2: Happy Lifestyle 39

Mother Nature's Answer 3: Happy Relationships 59

Appendix A: Essential Oils for Treating Different
Mood Conditions 85

Appendix B: Essential Oils and Their Emotional Impact 91

Acknowledgments 105

Notes 107

Recommended Resources 119

About the Author 123

About the Cowriter 124

Nutrition and Depression: The Effects of dōTERRA's
Lifelong Vitality Pack® on Depression and Anxiety 127

Introduction

Overcoming Depression Naturally

Everyone wants to be happy. Yet more and more people around the world today are unhappy. Something clearly has gone wrong, and our immediate attention is needed to overcome it. We owe a better life to our families, our friends and coworkers, our communities, and ourselves.

Depression is one of the largest problems our world faces. The World Health Organization (WHO) rates it as the leading cause of disability worldwide and reports that it's a major contributor to the global burden of disease. It's expensive, debilitating, and deadly.[1] In the United States, 25 percent of the population suffers from depression.[2] The number is somewhat lower in the United Kingdom, where about 20 percent of adults experience anxiety and/or depression.[3] Statistics are no better elsewhere. Approximately 350 million people worldwide are affected by depression. That's one in twenty individuals experiencing a depressive symptom each year. Global estimates show that one million people on average commit suicide each year; that's approximately 3,000 deaths per day resulting from symptoms of depression.[4] This mental health trend is not expected to change.

2 · ESSENTIALLY HAPPY

None of us wants to be counted as a negative statistic like this.

Clinical depression is described as persistent feelings of sadness or irritable mood; pronounced changes in sleep, appetite, and energy; difficulty thinking, concentrating, and remembering; physical slowing—or conversely, agitation; lack of interest in, and pleasure taken from activities that once were enjoyed; feelings of guilt, worthlessness, hopelessness, and emptiness; recurrent thoughts of death or suicide; and persistent physical symptoms that do not respond to treatment, such as headaches, digestive disorders, and chronic pain. When symptoms of depression become severe, people's lives become limited and narrow. Individuals with depression have so little energy they often cannot even get out of bed. It's a terrible and unfair state of being.

Several factors can contribute to depression. These include chemical imbalances and the experience of major chronic stress and trauma. Underlying biochemical and psychological issues may influence an individual to become depressed. Stressful events, such as mourning, loss of a job, or the breakup of a significant relationship can also trigger depression.

Depression is typically diagnosed on the basis of symptoms that can be mild, moderate, or severe. Although it is generally described as a chemical imbalance, in fact only a complex constellation of possible causes can explain such an imbalance. There are millions, even billions, of chemical reactions happening in our bodies every day that make up the dynamic system that's responsible for our moods, perceptions, and experiences of our lives. This whole system needs to be optimized. Science still has much to learn about the holistic biology of depression.

Researchers have identified genes that make some people more vulnerable to low moods, and can explain how different individuals are likely to respond to drug treatments.[5] But even though scientists know more than ever about how the brain regulates mood, our understanding of the functional biology of depression is still lacking. Certainly the ability to effectively treat it through medical means is lacking, otherwise the problem of depression would be shrinking.

We need alternatives—or means within our own control that complement our drugs.

Antidepressant medications are the most common form of treatment for depression at present. The annual costs of antidepressants in the United States for 1985 were $240 million. More recently, that number has jumped to $12 billion. Since 1995, 27 million people have taken them. Even though antidepressants are widely prescribed by doctors—in 2011 they were the most frequently dispensed drug—in fact, cases of depression continue to increase, suggesting that antidepressant medications are not working as well as expected.[6]

There currently is a crisis of confidence in antidepressants among many physicians.[7] In his 1981 book *Overcoming Depression*, Andrew Stanway, M.D., pointed out, "If antidepressant drugs were really as effective as they are made out to be, surely hospital admission rates for depression would have fallen over the twenty years they've been available. Alas, this has not happened. . . . Many trials have found that tricyclics are only marginally more effective than placebos, and some have even found that they are not as effective as dummy tablets."[8]

Some twenty years more after these words were written, researchers looked through the results of seventy-five studies in which participants were randomly selected to receive either a placebo or an antidepressant. The results revealed that people's responses to placebo increased along with their responses to antidepressant medication, calling into question the efficacy of the drugs.[9] The fact that studies continue to demonstrate variable successes with a placebo indicates a need for continuing research into how antidepressants are tested, and against which standards.

Existing drugs are effective in only about 50 percent of patients with depression.[10] Furthermore, these drugs can take three to four weeks before their beneficial effects manifest. And as with all drugs, there are a number of potential unwanted side effects.

While 50 percent relief of symptoms may sound impressive as a test result, it's not good enough for real life. Not your life. Not my life. Not anyone's life. If you are struggling with depression, you want relief. You want complete elimination of your symptoms and complete restoration of your psychological and social capabilities. Why shouldn't you get relief?

If a medication cannot achieve absolute elimination of your symptoms, then other avenues should be explored. For depression, these avenues are the remedies that Mother Nature has provided for us, which include nutrition, exercise, and stress reduction, among other things. Natural remedies, like the ones you'll find in this book, which have minimal side effects, if any, and contribute positively to overall health and well-being, should be part of everyone's life.

Much of what mainstream antidepressants do centers on the body's ability to create and maintain appropriate levels of serotonin, a brain chemical. This is what Prozac®, Zoloft®, Paxil®, and other selective serotonin reuptake inhibitors (SSRIs) are designed for. SSRIs block absorption of serotonin in the brain, thus enhancing brain cells' ability to communicate with one another—in the process, boosting mood. Along with SSRIs, however, can come side effects like nausea, nervousness, dizziness, drowsiness, lack of libido, insomnia, weight gain or loss, headache, dry mouth, vomiting, and diarrhea, often leading patients to choose to go untreated.[11]

Simon N. Young, former editor in chief of the *Journal of Psychiatry and Neuroscience*, has done significant research into the effects of serotonin levels on mood and overall health. He advocates finding ways to elevate levels without pharmacological methods, emphasizing the relationship between folate and serotonin.[12] As far back as 1962, studies of patients with depression found a high incidence among them of folic acid deficiency.

During the past two decades, research has begun to point to poor nutrition as a factor in the development of depression. Lack of essential fatty acids, imbalanced homocysteine levels, imbalanced serotonin levels caused by lack of amino acids, blood sugar imbalance, imbalanced levels of the nutrients chromium and vitamin D, and food intolerances are particularly problematic.[13] If we are undernourished, the biochemistry of our brains cells is affected.

In 2014, I designed a research study to determine whether or not high-quality nutritional supplements could be considered an adequate treatment for depression. For the study, I selected a comprehensive, multicomponent dietary supplement, Lifelong Vitality Pack®, manufactured by dōTERRA® and formulated to contain vitamins and minerals, essential fatty acids, polyphenols, and other nutritional energy cofactors previously shown to support optimal health. Participants were individuals diagnosed with depression who were not currently taking antidepressant medication. They took the dietary supplements twice daily during a period of sixty days and experienced significant relief.

It's no secret that I use essential oils. As an emotional counselor, I have found them to be effective adjuncts to my healing work with clients troubled by different problems. My family, friends, and I use them to effectively overcome physical, mental, and emotional ailments, finding that the body, mind, and spirit really are one. My passion for essential oils led me to research nonmedical treatments for depression and write this book for you.

What are Mother Nature's ways of helping us be happy? Natural approaches such as eating well, avoiding toxins, exercising, managing stress, and engaging in healthy relationships, are the foundation for good mental health. As the world has changed in the past few decades, our food has become less nourishing; our air, food, and water supplies have become more toxic from contamination with heavy metals, pesticides, hormones, and synthetic chemical additives; we have become sedentary; we're overwhelmed by technology and unending mental stimulation; and we've become more isolated and disconnected. It's no wonder we're feeling moody and anxious. Human biology is ill-equipped to handle the contemporary lifestyle.

Bottom line: The answer is to consider if jumping straight into taking drugs is really necessary. Maybe a better answer would be to get healthy so that you don't need to take drugs or so your efforts can complement your medicine.

The purpose of *Essentially Happy* is to suggest tools and techniques to sustain and improve your mood no matter where you fall on the scale of happiness and depression. I decided to ask the question: "How do we elevate mood and maintain happiness?" and then see what inspiring answers are available from Mother Nature. She had three simple ones.
- **Answer 1:** Happy nutrition
- **Answer 2:** Happy lifestyle
- **Answer 3:** Happy relationships

As common sense would tell you, it's best—easiest—to take steps to be happy before your mood sinks so low that you feel entirely hopeless and lack the energy to move forward and feel better. It's not enough to advise you, for instance, to do vigorous aerobic exercise three times a week. Although this could bring you

50 percent relief from depressive symptoms, if you can't see your way clear to get out of your bed, you're not going to be able to do it. Instead you have to begin where you are, with slow walks and gentle stretching, and then build up.

Some people report a dramatic shift when they change their diets, others when they improve their sleep habits and reduce stress, others by ending conflict with their relatives. If you're feeling down or blue, please try these suggestions and see if they work for you, too.

You deserve to be happy.

Rebecca Linder Hintze, M.Sc.
September 2014

Mother Nature's Answer 1

HAPPY NUTRITION

Our physical health has an impact on our moods. If we're in good health physically, we feel energetic and ready to take on the world. If we feel unwell physically, we feel like resting and retreating from the world. Generally, the more severe an underlying health condition becomes and the longer it lasts, the more fatigued we feel and the greater likelihood there is that our thoughts will be blue and pessimistic. We perhaps feel disappointed or even worried that we cannot do the activities we want to do. Today, depression is viewed as a marker for discovering deeper, underlying conditions.

Our mental and emotional health can be adversely affected by everything from food sensitivities and yeast overgrowth in our guts, to poor liver function, systemic inflammation, thyroid disorders, and more. It is important, therefore, to take the whole body into consideration whenever we're trying to manage depression. Mother Nature's first answer for mood elevation is to nourish the body with well-balanced meals from high-quality food sources. With proper nutrition, we can resolve or reduce the symptoms of some of these health issues and diseases. Food is a factor that is often overlooked in the pursuit of optimal physical and mental health.

Depression is a multifaceted condition, so it may take a combination of efforts to manage or overcome it. Solutions range from exercising to reducing stress and talking to someone or writing about your feelings. If you're experiencing persistent sadness or you have thoughts of harming yourself, it is important to bring your condition to the attention of a healthcare provider. There are individuals for whom antidepressant medication is helpful to balance the brain chemistry. That being said, no matter what else you do, adjusting your nutritional intake to improve your physical health is a good first step. Please be advised that it is never a good idea to stop taking prescribed medication suddenly and without professional counsel. Your healthcare provider can help you to assess your options and devise a treatment plan, or refer you to a specialist.

In treating depression naturally, we should look for ways to support the brain, liver, gastrointestinal tract, and thyroid in particular. If any of these organs is malfunctioning, it is likely to produce a whole constellation of symptoms, from the subtle to the severe, including symptoms of depression. Feeding ourselves in order to nourish these individual organs, as well as cleaning up conditions and imbalances that prevent them from functioning optimally, and using gifts from Mother Nature may enable us to eradicate our depression altogether.

Mother Nature in her glory provided us with organic, pesticide-free, antibiotic-free, hormone-free, non-genetically modified (non-GMO) foods—both plants and animals. If we stay as close as possible to the goodness of her food supply when we're making food choices, and eat only clean, unrefined and unprocessed foods, we can greatly enhance our well-being. Ideally, that means clean water, fresh organic fruits and vegetables, grass-fed meats (and dairy), wild fish, and free-range poultry (and eggs). Do the best you can to make good, clean choices.

In our present world, much of the soil in which we grow our food lacks nutrients. For a variety of reasons, it has become depleted. To ensure we're getting adequate amounts of vitamins and minerals, even those of which we only need trace amounts, being well-nourished may require supplementation. Try it and see if it works for you. Let your own body and mind guide you.

Eating a well-balanced diet lays the foundation for happiness.

THE BRAIN-MOOD CONNECTION

There are millions, even billions, of chemical reactions going on in your brain and body all the time that make up the complex and dynamic system that is responsible for your moods and perceptions, and influences how you experience life. Scientific understanding of the biology of the brain is limited, yet growing rapidly through continued research. To date, this much is known for sure: Your individual brain cells, or *neurons*, release chemicals that transmit impulses to other neurons inside your brain and to more distant nerve cells located throughout your body's muscles, organs, and tissues. These chemical messengers regulate your physiology. Among other things, they make your heart beat and your stomach digest food.

There are two kinds of neurotransmitters: *excitatory* and *inhibitory*. Both types are necessary for our survival. Excitatory neurotransmitters stimulate the brain. Inhibitory neurotransmitters calm the brain. When the brain is overstimulated or the stimulation goes on too long, as happens when we're under severe or persistent stress, inhibitory brain chemicals become depleted. When this happens, we lose the ability to balance activity with rest, which puts enormous strain on the body and brain. At such a time, we can also become depleted of excitatory neurotransmitters, making it hard to function or take action, and leading to a series of low-energy symptoms.

Interestingly, while more than 100 neurotransmitters regulate communication in the brain, six explain most of human behavior: serotonin, dopamine, norepinephrine, acetylcholine, gamma-aminobutyric acid (GABA), and glutamate. Of these, serotonin, GABA, and dopamine are inhibitory. Generally, that is. Under some conditions, dopamine can also be stimulating.

Norepinephrine, acetylcholine, and glutamate are excitatory neurotransmitters.

Imbalances of these six neurotransmitters are associated with different diseases. For example, low **serotonin** levels are connected with depression, lack of sleep, and impulsive behavior. The rarer condition of high serotonin leads to confusion, agitation, heart palpitations, and hallucinations.

An excess of **dopamine** is associated with schizophrenia, and a deficiency of dopamine with, among other things, stiff, rigid, achy muscles; poor balance; and "brain fog."

A disproportionate amount of **norepinephrine** (aka noradrenaline), or of **acetylcholine,** is associated with a lack of focus, irritability, and jumpiness. Norepinephrine plays a key role in the fight-or-flight stress response that is so damaging if it persists in our lives. High levels can be associated with joy at times, and low levels with fibromyalgia and chronic fatigue.

An imbalance between **glutamate** and **GABA** can contribute to anxiety, restlessness, or ADHD-like distraction of the kind we experience when we work too long on our computers. Glutamate is stimulating. If the effects of glutamate are not tempered by GABA, its presence will eventually damage and kill off your brain cells.

On the other hand, if there is a glutamate deficiency, you may experience insomnia, low energy, and mental exhaustion. **GABA** is calming. It is involved with sleep, relaxation, anxiety regulation, and muscle function.

When we are properly nourished, this biochemical system is better regulated.

WHAT CAUSES AN IMBALANCE OF BRAIN CHEMICALS?

Neurotransmitters are made within the brain cells. Anything that prevents these cells from making a certain kind of chemical creates a deficiency.

The primary cause of low levels of neurotransmitters is nutritional deficiency. Your brain makes these important signaling chemicals from the amino acids you ingest from your food.

Another root cause of deficiencies of neurotransmitters is anything that damages neurons. This could include both environmental factors, like exposure to toxins, and emotional factors, such as the stress response.

Genetics play a role, too. Your genes may cause your brain cells to produce either too much or too little of a given neurotransmitter. The relatively new field of epigenetics is studying how environmental conditions, including exogenous ones such as nutrition and pollution, and endogenous ones such as thoughts and emotions, can flip on/off switches in genes and alter our predisposition to certain health issues. Certain cognitive diseases with a genetic link, such as Alzheimer's disease, relate to the physiological impairment of brain cells.

Overuse of a specific neurotransmitter can lead to its depletion, causing an imbalance. In our increasingly volatile, uncertain, and complicated world, many of us are challenged to remain calm. An almost unending stress response catches up with us if our neurons keep firing off the chemicals that make us biologically capable of responding to immediate danger. We can burn out, just like a piece of electrical equipment that has overheated.

Sometimes imbalance is caused by a problem on the other side of the signaling process—a problem not with the production or release of a chemical messenger, but how it is received. It's like sending an email, only to have it bounce back from someone's inbox. The receptors in cells that are supposed to bind with neurotransmitters may not be available or functioning properly for some reason. In this case, the unused neurotransmitters build up in the body.

Since your body forms these important brain chemicals itself, foods whose nutrients may be used as building blocks for manufacturing them are vital to your well-being. While you may not be able to compensate for every kind of physiological damage to your neurons that happens in your lifetime, there are some measures you can take day by day to ensure that the damage to your brain cells is minimal and that your brain has what it needs to function optimally.

Simply put, you should defend your brain and also work to strengthen its capacities. The nutritional composition of every meal you eat matters a great deal, as it has the potential to affect your physical and mental health and your mood.

NUTRIENTS THAT PROMOTE BRAIN HEALTH

Eating nutrition-packed foods is vital to the transmission of information from cell to cell. In order for the body to make neurotransmitters, it must gather the ingredients they are composed of along with the correct nutritional cofactors to manufacture them. This allows for the production of the neurotransmitter to be efficient and effective. A partial list of nutrients required for synthesis of neurotransmitters includes amino acids (tryptophan, tyrosine, glutamine), minerals (zinc, copper, iron, magnesium), and B-vitamins (B6, B12, folic acid).

Let's look at each of these in turn.

Amino Acids (Tryptophan, Tyrosine, Glutamine)

According to the Biology Project at the University of Arizona, "Amino acids play central roles both as building blocks of proteins and as intermediates in metabolism.... The chemical properties of the amino acids of proteins determine the biological activity of the protein. Proteins not only catalyze all (or most) of the reactions in living cells, they control virtually all cellular process. In addition, proteins contain within their amino acid sequences the necessary information to determine how that protein will fold into a three-dimensional structure, and the stability of the resulting structure."[1]

Twenty amino acids are needed to sustain our lives. Of these, our bodies can produce ten: alanine, asparagine, aspartic acid, cysteine, glutamic acid, glutamine, glycine, proline, serine, and tyrosine. The rest must come through our food supply. Because it is essential that our diets contain them, these second ten are known as *essential amino acids.* They are arginine, histidine, isoleucine, leucine, lysine, methionine, phenylalanine, threonine, tryptophan, and valine.[2]

The brain uses the essential amino acid **tryptophan** to make the neurotransmitters serotonin, melatonin, tryptamine, and indoleanine, which are antidepressants and regulate blood sugar and blood pressure. Tryptophan is also necessary for the production of niacin, a B vitamin involved in the manufacture of nerves. The cofactors necessary for tryptophan to be converted to niacin are B6, riboflavin, and iron.

Dietary sources of tryptophan are: cheese, chicken, eggs, fish, milk, peanuts, pumpkin seeds, soy, sesame seeds, and turkey.

Tyrosine is a nonessential amino acid involved in the production of dopamine and of the stress hormones epinephrine and norepinephrine. It helps in the function of the adrenal gland, the pituitary gland, and the thyroid gland.

Dietary sources of tyrosine are: almonds, avocadoes, bananas, cheese, chicken, cottage cheese, fish, lima beans, milk, peanuts, pumpkin seeds, sesame seeds, soy, turkey, and yogurt.

Glutamine is a nonessential amino acid that is critical for the immune system, the brain, and digestion. It is usually abundant but when the body is stressed, injured, or ill, as levels of the stress hormone cortisol go up, more glutamine is needed.

Dietary sources of glutamine are: cabbage, cottage cheese, beef, milk, pork, poultry, raw spinach, raw parsley, ricotta cheese, and yogurt.

Caution: Because of the potential for side effects and adverse interactions with medications, anyone considering taking a glutamine supplement should do so only under the supervision of a knowledgeable healthcare provider.

Minerals (Zinc, Copper, Iron, Magnesium)

A mineral is an inorganic solid compound. Several are essential for our diets, but we're only going to look at four in this section, starting with zinc. Adequate levels of **zinc** are necessary for the function of the parts of the brain cells that release serotonin and glutamate. If we have a deficiency and serotonin production goes down, this deficiency may reveal itself in the form of irritability and depression, among other things.[3]

Interestingly, although zinc is a cofactor in 300 enzymatic reactions, the highest amount of it in the body is present in the brain.[4]

Dietary sources of zinc are: baked beans, beef, cashews, cheese, chicken, chickpeas, milk, oatmeal, pork, and especially shellfish (oysters, crab, lobster). Vegetarians need to be particularly mindful to get enough zinc because the best sources are meat proteins.

Copper is a trace mineral whose levels fluctuate inversely with zinc. When zinc is prevalent, copper levels fall. When zinc levels fall, as they may do in cases of adrenal burnout from ongoing stress, copper accumulates. Copper stimulates production of the neurotransmitters epinephrine, norepinephrine, and dopamine. Interestingly, many people have excessive copper in their systems today because of environmental sources, such as cookware, water pipes, and pesticides.[5]

Dietary sources of copper are: beans, chocolate, grains, nuts, and seeds.

Iron carries oxygen throughout the bloodstream. It also helps the muscles store oxygen. It is part of many enzymes, substances that aid in digestion and are involved in many other cellular reactions. When levels of iron are low, anxiety, depression, and other psychological disturbances become possible.[6]

Dietary sources of iron are: apricots, beef liver, broccoli, chicken liver, chickpeas, clams, green pepper, kidney beans, lima beans, mussels, potatoes, pumpkin seeds, sardines, sesame seeds, spinach, turkey, and wheat germ.

Magnesium protects the brain from the body's own toxic waste products, such as ammonia. It is a cofactor in 300 enzyme systems that regulate diverse biochemical reactions, including muscle and nerve functions, and the regulation of blood sugar and blood pressure. A deficiency causes migraines, poor sleep, ADHD, anxiety, and depression.[7]

Here's an interesting fact: Plants use magnesium to make chlorophyll, which turns them green, so leafy green vegetables contain oodles of it.

Dietary sources of magnesium are: blackstrap molasses, beet greens, broccoli, collard greens, green beans, halibut, salmon, spinach, and Swiss chard.

B Vitamins (B6, B12, Folic Acid)

A vitamin is an organic compound and vital nutrient that the body needs in small quantities. When it comes to brain health, enhancing mood, and overcoming depression, the B vitamins are particularly significant.

The B vitamins are critical for producing brain chemicals. According to the Mayo Clinic, older adults, vegetarians, and people with malabsorption issues in the gut and liver can have trouble getting adequate amounts of B6, B12, and folic acid (folate).[8]

According to the National Institutes of Health, "The body needs **vitamin B6** for more than 100 enzyme reactions involved in metabolism. Vitamin B6 is also involved in brain development during pregnancy and infancy as well as immune function."[9]

Dietary sources of B6 are: bananas, beef, chicken, potatoes, salmon, spinach, sunflower seeds, sweet potatoes, tuna, and turkey.

Vitamin B12 is involved in energy production and is a cofactor of DNA, the genetic material involved in cell replication. If you eat meat, it's hard to become deficient in B12, because the body is capable of storing it. However, low levels are known to result from malabsorption, and alcohol can leech it from the body. If it is absent, serotonin production may be interrupted, leading to mood disorders and other issues.

Dietary sources of B12 are: beef, eggs, lamb, milk, poultry, salmon, sardines, shrimp, tuna, and yogurt.

Folic acid is a B vitamin recognized for playing a critical role in the development of the fetal brain during pregnancy. In adults, it helps prevent the buildup of homocysteine, which can lead to inflammation; and it supports red blood cell production, which helps prevent iron deficiency.[10]

Dietary sources of folic acid are: asparagus, black beans, broccoli, calf's liver, garbanzo beans, kidney beans, lentils, navy beans, pinto beans, romaine lettuce, spinach, and turnip greens.

Omega-3 Fatty Acids

The entire body depends on fat to function—it's present in every single cell—and the brain is especially dependent on one kind of fat: **omega-3**.

According to the Cleveland clinic, omega-3 fatty acids are great for heart health: They lower the risk of sudden death from heart arrhythmia, reduce blood clot formation, inhibit the growth of plaque, decrease triglycerides (produced in the liver), lower blood pressure, and have anti-inflammatory properties.[11]

Omega-3 fatty acid, in the form of alpha-linolenic acid (ALA), is present in plants, such as flax and chia. Flaxseeds and chia seeds are widely available in supermarkets and health food stores. Incorporating these into your diet offers the benefits of providing flavor and fiber, and these seeds are good for the body, especially the heart. When they are liquefied into the form of oil, as they are for supplementation, they destabilize quickly on the shelf—so they must be kept refrigerated and used before expiration.

The best marine sources of omega-3s are: deep-water fish such as tuna, salmon, mackerel, trout, and sardines, which pack on fat to survive the cold temperature of the water. It's actually the algae that fish eat that makes them great sources of omega-3. Some supplements are made from krill oil, which is packed with omega-3 because krill eat a lot of phytoplankton, the plant they get their omega-3s from in the ocean. Two kinds of omega-3 fat are present in fish: eicosapentaenoic acid (EPA) and docosahexaenoic acid (DHA).

Some omega-3 supplements contain astaxanthin, a powerful antioxidant that preserves its freshness. Astaxanthin belongs to a class of phytochemicals known as terpenes that are found in microalgae, yeast, salmon, trout, shrimp, crayfish, and in some cases, birds. It's classified as a xanthophyll and has a yellow pigment. Bottom line, astaxanthin is an important addition to some omega-3 supplements because it helps preserve quality and efficacy. Among other things, astaxanthin supports dementia and Alzheimer's, acts as a natural sunscreen, and can boost the immune system. Krill oil naturally contains astaxanthin.

Others sources of omega-3s are: grass-fed cattle that graze on green pastures, and eggs from free-range chickens.[12] Both are beneficial.

For brain health and to bring some relief from depression, the omega-3 fatty acid you want to consume is DHA. DHA accounts for up to 97 percent of the omega-3 fatty acids in the brain, and ensures that the cells in the brain and other parts of the nervous system develop and function properly. Interestingly, DHA is found in human breast milk.

TWO SURPRISING GOOD-MOOD FOODS

Do you like Italian food or Indian food? Then you'll love these good-mood foods.

Garlic. Garlic has many benefits, not the least of which is its high concentration of antioxidants and its ability to lower blood pressure and cholesterol. In terms of mood elevation, there has been promising research. In the 1990s, Dr. Gilles Fillion of the Pasteur Institute found that garlic affects the release of serotonin.[13] He said, "I suspect garlic is anti-stress, anti-anxiety, and acts as a sort of antidepressant like Prozac, although with a much milder effect."[14]

Turmeric. Do you like to eat curry? If so, you're in luck. Turmeric, the yellow root that is the main ingredient in curry, contains high levels of curcumin, which has long been known to reduce inflammation. A recent randomized, controlled study of women with depression in India also found that turmeric is more effective at treating depression than Prozac—and without unpleasant side effects.[15]

ESSENTIAL OILS FOR OVERCOMING DEPRESSION

To balance mood swings and get clarity:

Oil protocol: In a glass roller bottle, blend equal parts frankincense and wild orange.

Application: Roll and rub between hands and inhale; apply to bottoms of feet and chest three to four times a day.

DRINK WATER AND FEEL BETTER

Dehydration is often overlooked as a possible culprit for complicating mental health issues. The body is made up of 95 percent water, so we need to drink water every day in order to live. Electrolytes—mineral molecules that dissolve in water—such as potassium, calcium, and sodium, are critical to our well-being. When we don't have enough water, we often feel lethargic and grumpy, and we can get headaches and have all kinds of other health complications.

We can mistake thirst for hunger, and it is not uncommon to crave salty foods when we're slightly dehydrated because the body is innately intelligent and "knows" that salt enables us to retain fluids. We might be tempted to get out a bag of chips instead of drinking a glass or two of water, but the water is where we should always start.

If you believe you have been dehydrated for a while, for a period of time (try thirty days) make it a point to drink half your body weight in ounces over the course of your waking day. That means, if you are a 160-pound individual, drink eighty ounces of plain water—or ten eight-ounce glasses divided one per hour over a ten-hour stretch.

For the purpose of hydration, soda, sweet lemonade, coffee, tea, and flavored drinks do not count as water; they can actually complicate healing because they contain sugar and caffeine, which are two of the top substances we should avoid.

FOUR "BAD BOYS" MOTHER NATURE DOESN'T WANT YOU TO PLAY WITH

When we're feeling blue, we often turn to the wrong substances, trying to get a pick-me-up. That's because we are predisposed biologically to respond to the presence of fat, salt, and sugar. Our ancestors craved these foods because Mother Nature programmed us to want them as a survival instinct in the harsh conditions of the wild. Of course, now that we are surrounded by plenty in our supermarkets, we need to be wary of them. In the book *Salt, Sugar, Fat,* Michael Moss reveals how the food industry has learned to push our buttons so we make poor choices at the checkout counter. Don't let yourself be manipulated into eating too much of these foods.

Processed Food

Processed foods are laden with salt, sugar, and fat and are lacking good nutritional content. Mounting research reports that poor nutrition is directly related to depression.

According to a recent study from the University of Las Palmas de Gran Canaria and the University of Granada, eating commercially baked goods (cakes, croissants, doughnuts, and so on) and greasy fast food (hamburgers, hotdogs, and pizza) can be linked to depression.[16] The report of this six-year study headed by Almudena Sanchez-Villegas was published in *Public Health Nutrition*. It revealed that consumers of fast food (compared with those who eat little or no fast food) are 51 percent more likely to develop depression than those who don't. Furthermore, the more fast foods people consume, the more at risk they are for depression.[17]

With depression, it is often difficult to determine which comes first. Did having chronic headaches lead to depression, for instance, or did depression lead to chronic headaches? Likewise, did poor eating habits cause someone's depression, or did a fast-food habit take hold in this person as a means of coping—however ineffectively—with their depression?

Sugar

Everyone loves sugar, and sweets can help us feel good temporarily when we eat them, but they are a temporary mood fix at best. That's because sugar is absorbed quickly into the bloodstream, which causes an initial surge of energy that makes us feel "high." Soon, that rush wears off, however, as the body increases insulin production to remove the sugar from the bloodstream. In the end, we're left feeling tired and lower in energy than when we started.

Sugar and carbohydrates from sources like grains, which are quickly digested, contribute to chronic inflammation, which disrupts the body's immune system. Plants are so high in fiber that their carbs are digested more slowly and do not produce the same inflammatory response. Acute inflammation is a natural response that the body employs temporarily to heal the body after an injury. White blood cells rush to the site of damage, causing swelling as they initiate repairs. But when the immune system begins to respond to everything with an inflammatory response, it wreaks havoc throughout the body, including the brain.

Sugar suppresses the production of a key hormone called brain-derived neurotrophic factor (BDNF), which promotes the growth and ongoing health of neurons, and plays a vital role in memory. BDNF levels are critically low in people with depression. Some research suggests that these low levels may actually be a causative factor in depression.[18]

Sugar is hidden in pretty much every processed food because the food industry knows that this makes us like such products. And interestingly, every kind of sugar produces the exact same metabolic response in the body. It's doesn't matter if you are eating table sugar, honey, molasses, or fructose. Sugar is sugar is sugar is sugar. Some sugary foods are entirely devoid of nutrition, making them a terrible choice nutritionally speaking; whereas other sugary foods (fruit, molasses, honey) do offer some nutritional value that makes them better choices, for the most part. Rule of thumb: Avoid hidden sugars and choose your "poison" wisely. Read labels!

Sugar can damage our nervous system and tax the liver. Excess glucose in the bloodstream oxidizes and forms advanced glycation end products (AGEs). These degenerate the brain. Sugar also kills the symbiotic bacteria in the gut that produce B vitamins for us[19] Those B vitamins play a major role in brain functions. So clearly, sugar should be avoided at all costs.

Caffeine

Some people drink coffee and other beverages that contain caffeine (tea, soda, and hot chocolate) to help boost their energy levels. The problem is that caffeine has been shown to diminish serotonin in the brain.[22] When serotonin is suppressed, it's easy to become depressed and feel irritable. Among other things, caffeine keeps you awake, possibly leading to insomnia, stress, and anxiety. Remember, you need to sleep well to be in a positive mood.

Caffeine is also a diuretic—meaning, it makes you need to urinate more often. Even mild dehydration can contribute to poor health and depression.

Alcohol

People often drink alcohol to ease stress and anxiety. Unfortunately, the feel-good effects are temporary and can cause additional anxiety and stress once the high the alcohol provided has worn off. Alcohol is a diuretic, so drinking alcohol requires a compensatory increase in water consumption to keep the body well and balanced.

Alcohol is a known depressant and can disrupt balance in the brain, affecting our thoughts, feelings, actions—even our long-term mental health—if we keep drinking it. This is partly due to the way alcohol affects the neurotransmission process in the brain and partly due to the fact that it is toxic to the liver. As liver function diminishes, we begin to feel sicker.

LIVER DISEASE AND DEPRESSION

The liver serves so many vital functions that it's a bit like a one-man band playing many different instruments simultaneously. Beside the brain, it's the most complicated organ in the entire body: It makes bile to emulsify fat for digestion. It makes and breaks down hormones, including cholesterol, estrogen, and testosterone. It regulates blood sugar. It filters food, alcohol, drugs, and environmental toxins: either letting them pass into the bloodstream, or breaking them down into byproducts that the body can excrete, or storing them. It can be damaged without any major overt signs; however, as its capacity further diminishes, you gradually feel worse.

Depression may indicate that the liver is having trouble performing its tasks for one of many possible reasons: It could, for example, be overloaded by poisonous substances, or infected with a strain of hepatitis, or so scarred by cirrhosis that blood flow and nutrient absorption are blocked. If you're feeling down, consider detoxifying the liver by avoiding alcohol, hydrating, eating fruits and vegetables (especially broccoli), and staying away from chemicals in your environment—no paint fumes, no pesticides, no dyes, no perfumes, no household cleaners, and so on. Give the liver a chance to rest and heal, and you may find your spirits being lifted.

NATURAL REMEDIES FOR LIVER HEALTH

The following are natural remedies that health experts recommend for supporting healthy liver function.

S-adenosylmethionine (SAMe)

Found throughout the body, SAMe is involved with producing serotonin, melatonin, and dopamine. It runs in shorter supply when the liver becomes unable to process B vitamins.[21] In laboratory tests, patients given 1,600 milligrams of SAMe per day showed significant improvement in liver function.[22] According to WebMD, there is no established ideal dose for depression; experts recommend taking 400 to 1,600 milligrams daily.[23]

Zinc Supplements

If you have inflammation, then zinc may get sequestered in the liver. Take 50 milligrams daily (no more) to make it more available.

Milk Thistle *(Silymarin)*

Take 420 milligrams daily. People with an allergy to ragweed or daisies should avoid it, since the plants are close cousins.[24] Many people with depression are suffering from a gut condition, such as dysbiosis (an imbalance of intestinal bacteria) or a yeast overgrowth. Milk thistle helps the liver to filter toxins, such as dead bacteria and yeast, from the blood stream. *Caution: If you're taking necessary medications, milk thistle may impede their functioning by causing them to break down too quickly.*

ESSENTIAL OILS FOR SUPPORTING THE LIVER

To lift and calm your mood:

Oil protocol: Mix equal parts of each oil in a glass roller bottle: juniper berry, geranium, thyme, and helichrysum.

Application: Apply topically over the liver twice a day and drink a lot of water.

THE GUT-BRAIN CONNECTION

If we want to improve our moods, another factor to consider alongside nutrition is the relationship between the digestive system and the brain. Our gastrointestinal (GI) tracts and our brains are in constant communication with one another via the vagus nerve. In fact, they are so responsive that a traumatic brain injury can cause gastrointestinal distress.[25] This gut-brain link is essential to understanding the mechanisms of depression.

Technically known as the enteric nervous system, the neurons that line the walls of the digestive tract running from the throat all the way to the anus, have been termed the *second brain*. According to Michael Gershon who wrote the book *The Second Brain*, the "signaling in the gut as part of our physiological stress response" (think butterflies before a big date or an important exam) is only one example of how the gut affects our moods.[26]

The gut uses thirty neurotransmitters.[27] Whenever something goes awry down there, in the brain below the belly button, our state of mind changes. "There's a two-way street between what's going on in the gut and what's going on in the brain," Linda A. Lee, the director of the Johns Hopkins Integrative Medicine and Digestive Center, is quoted as saying in a March 2014 article in the *Washington Post*.[28]

Recent research is finding that gut bacteria affects brain activity. Improving the ratio of helpful gut flora to harmful gut flora is another avenue to consider in treating depression. At the University of California, Los Angeles, researchers studied healthy women who had not demonstrated either gastrointestinal symptoms or psychological symptoms. Half the group was given probiotics *(B. animalis, S. thermophilus, L. bulgaricus, and L. lactis)* twice a day for four weeks. The other half was given none. When the women underwent functional magnetic resonance imaging (fMRI), activity in regions of the brain that control processing of emotions was clearly affected by the intake of the probiotics.[29]

FOOD SENSITIVITIES AND SYSTEMIC INFLAMMATION

Food sensitivities are a root cause of systemic inflammation. Dairy products, legumes, and grains tend to be the most inflammatory foods in our diets. Some of the population does not possess enzymes capable of breaking down the proline proteins in grains, especially gluten and gliadin. The saponins in legumes, and the lactose and the casein in dairy are also problematic for many people. When undigested particles of these foods cross through the permeable walls of the intestines into the bloodstream, the body treats the particles like foreign invaders and sends an immune response with cytokines. That response produces inflammation.

Whenever particles penetrate the gut wall that should not cross through, the condition is known as *leaky gut syndrome*. If the intestinal lining is damaged, it must be healed. You likely need to improve the way your food is being digested. Confer with a health practitioner to assess the underlying causes and address them.

Systemic inflammation can be caused by a number of factors. Having excess adipose (fat) tissue in the body is one factor. Adipose tissue releases a number of inflammatory factors, of which one is cytokine, a small protein important in cell signaling. Cytokines are proven to play a role in insulin resistance and increased risk for cardiovascular disease. They also cause inflammation within our brains when they pass through the blood-brain barrier. When cytokines cross into our hypothalamus and other parts of the brain that control mood, they can cause serious problems for us, including mood disorders. In a report in *Molecular Psychiatry*, Dr. J. Licinio explained that inflammatory cytokines play a role in major depression. These cytokines can be formed from a number of factors such as; stress, body weight, sleep, food intake, and body temperature.[30]

Celiac disease is a genetic autoimmune disorder of the small intestine, involving a heightened inflammatory response to wheat protein; it often leads to vitamin deficiencies. People with celiac disease report much higher rates of depression then the average person. The only known effective treatment is a lifelong gluten-free diet.

Intolerance to fruit and milk sugars (fructose and lactose) has been linked to malabsorption of the essential amino acid tryptophan, which as we have discussed, may be linked to serotonin deficiency, clinical depression, anxiety, and ADHD.

DYSBIOSIS AND CANDIDA SYNDROME

We have symbiotic relationships with many of the bacteria that populate our intestines, such as *L. bulgaricus*, which help us to manufacture the B vitamins we need to sustain our lives. These bacteria are probiotic. Other bacteria, like *E. coli*, are deadly if they are not kept in check by our immune system, intestinal pH, and other, friendlier bacteria. When the number of bad bacteria exceeds a healthy proportion, the condition we face is known as *dysbiosis*.

Along with bacteria, the gut contains fungi, one of the most prevalent of which is the yeast called *Candida albicans*. Yeast that overgrows is a recognized culprit in many health disorders, and causes symptoms that include abdominal bloating, constipation or diarrhea (or both), fatigue, anxiety, fuzzy thinking, insomnia, mood swings, and depression, among others. In the book *Digestive Wellness*, Elizabeth Lipski, Ph.D., CCN, offers a comprehensive discussion of candida, saying that it is an underlying cause of food sensitivities.[31] Candida dysbiosis can result from taking antibiotics, birth control pills, and steroids, and consuming too much sugar and alcohol—which yeast thrives on. Another reason to avoid those bad boys!

NATURAL REMEDIES FOR DIGESTIVE HEALTH

If you believe that food sensitivities, inflammation, or dysbiosis (candida syndrome) may be an issue for you, remove triggering foods from your diet. Also take these steps:

- **Replenish your gut bacteria.** Take probiotics.
- **Eliminate sugary food from your diet.** Avoid fruit, alcohol, soda, grains, and potatoes.
- **Supplement with antioxidant nutrients.** To heal the lining of the gut, take vitamin A, vitamin C, and vitamin E, folic acid, selenium, and zinc.
- **Visit a healthcare professional.**

ESSENTIAL OILS FOR TREATING CANDIDA DYSBIOSIS

To heal an overgrowth of candida albicans:

Oil protocol: Take equal parts of therapeutic-grade (safe for internal use) oregano, melaleuca, thyme, and lemon internally (two drops of each) in a capsule two to three times a day with food.

Alternate daily dosing with taking a probiotic.

DEPRESSION AND THE THYROID GLAND

The thyroid gland produces and regulates hormones, including those for mood. Some symptoms of depression are associated with conditions that could indicate an underactive thyroid, such as low energy, low libido, weight gain, forgetfulness, and trouble sleeping. Women are significantly more likely to have low thyroid hormone production than men, and it's worth checking in with your doctor if you think this may be an issue for you, especially in mid-life (around the time of menopause) when changes are occurring in your endocrine system.

Clues that your thyroid may be sluggish are that your skin and hair become extremely brittle and you feel more sensitive than you formerly did to cold and heat.

NATURAL REMEDIES FOR THYROID HEALTH

First line of defense for hypothyroidism is to modify your diet.[32] Thyroid health is usually related to an immune system issue, so lifestyle and dietary modifications may be helpful.
- Reduce or eliminate caffeine and sugar.
- Stock up on omega-3 fats.
- Address underlying food sensitivities, such as intolerance to gluten.
- Reduce stress to heal adrenal fatigue.

ESSENTIAL OILS FOR LOW THYROID

To stimulate a sluggish thyroid gland:

Oil protocol: Dilute two drops each of clove, myrrh, and lemongrass oil in one tablespoon of carrier oil (coconut or almond or safflower).

Application: Apply this oil blend topically to the base of your throat (over the thyroid gland) and the soles of your feet.

TO BE HAPPY, TAKE VITAMIN, MINERAL, AND OMEGA-3 SUPPLEMENTS

While in graduate school, I conducted a study using nutritional supplements as a treatment for depression and found that the supplements had a significant and sustainable effect on mood in a short period of time. The outcomes suggested that poor nutrition plays a role in depression, and that quality supplementation may be a useful form of treatment for mood disorders.

This research constituted a preliminary investigation into the effects on people's moods of a potent nutritional supplement pack called Lifelong Vitality® (LLV), which is marketed for daily use by dōTERRA Corporation. This nutritional supplement pack contains vitamins and minerals, essential fatty acids, polyphenols, and other nutritional cofactors that support optimal health. The sixty-day study followed a single group of subjects diagnosed with anxiety or depression who were not currently taking any medication.

In some cases, having a deficiency of a certain vitamin, mineral, amino acid, or fatty acid can relate directly to your emotional well-being. Depression is a complex issue, however, that is not generally caused by just a single factor. Therefore supporting the body by providing it with balanced and adequate overall nutrition is a step in the right direction to promote healing. The impact of diet on depression was underestimated and not understood until recently. Today nutrition for mental health is a topic that merits further consideration and research.

PLANT-BASED MEDICINE

The art of plant medicine has been practiced for thousands of years in diverse cultures around the world with success. Any ingredient with an active therapeutic effect that is derived from a whole or a part of a plant can be considered plant medicine. So it's a term that loosely describes everything from herbs, to essential oils, and flower essences. But practitioners of one type of plant medicine usually do not have the training to understand another type.

Information provided here is being offered for inspiration and education. *Advisory: It is good to investigate potential interactions between herbs, essential oils, and pharmaceutical drugs. It is important to ensure that in taking multiple substances one does not neutralize one another or mix poorly.*

Herbs

Herbal medicine is practiced by naturopathic doctors, physicians trained in traditional Chinese medicine, and indigenous healers and shamans. A few of the best well-known herbal remedies that may be used to overcome depression can be found in your local health food store or almost any store that sells vitamin and mineral supplements.

For depression, two herbs that are commonly used are:
- St. John's wort
- Gingko biloba

Essential Oils

More recently than is the case with herbs, medical science began documenting exactly how depression and other mental health disorders can be improved or resolved with the use of essential oils. Well-respected doctors and researchers are now studying the effects of pure, therapeutic-grade essential oils from different parts of plants on infections, depression, and other ailments. Various essential oils not only support cellular communication and oxygenation of the blood, some also improve our neurochemistry by clearing receptor sites in the brain for neurotransmitters. This means essential oils can alter our perceptions. By supporting the production of neurotransmitters they make us feel happier.

Using therapeutic-grade essential oils that are tested and certified as being pure (safe enough to ingest) is easy. To begin, open any bottle and inhale its fragrance. Three effective applications of most high-quality essential oils include:

Aromatic use. Dispense several drops in hands, rub together, and inhale; or use a commercial water diffuser and breathe the molecules in vapor deeply throughout the day.

Topical use. Apply a few drops of the essential oil directly on the skin. *Caution: Sometimes dilution is indicated as necessary on the label.* We most frequently suggest applying to the bottoms of the feet, where absorption into the body systems happens quickly and effectively.

Internal use. Drip one or two drops of essential oil under the tongue, or mix into a glass of water and drink. You can also put drops in an empty veggie capsule and just swallow. (That's a better approach when the oil is particularly strong or acrid in taste.) Never swallow essential oils that have not been labeled as safe for ingestion.

All brands of essential oils are not alike; neither are plants. The essential oils that are best for mental health are the oils that have undergone extensive testing for purity by biochemists, using instruments such as mass spectrometry and gas chromatography. Not many companies complete these tests so it's important to qualify the essential oils you're using first, before using them to treat any health condition you may have.

You will find discussions of the properties of essential oils sprinkled throughout the rest the book as well as two appendices at the back of the book that can help you understand which essential oils may be appropriate for emotions and the health conditions you are experiencing.

In the next chapter, we'll look at Mother Nature's second answer for overcoming depression: embracing a natural lifestyle.

Mother Nature's Answer 2

Happy Lifestyle

We belong to Mother Nature, and come from Mother Nature, the ultimate source of life. For this reason, when we embrace a natural lifestyle, we find that life on Earth provides everything we need to live well and be happy. The modern world with its incredible conveniences often distances us from nature. But there is good evidence that something as simple as making contact regularly with green trees, grass, and plants can be mood enhancing. By adapting our activities to respond to our biology, we align our lifestyle with nature, and it can help us feel much better.

A defining characteristic of human nature is to be able to adapt to changing conditions and restore balance within mind and body; it is a tendency to move toward equilibrium. Anything that interrupts this process can disrupt your state of mind and your mood. Everything that facilitates it can elevate your mood and bring you greater peace of mind. If you embrace a natural lifestyle, the very rhythm of your existence will balance activity and rest, giving your mind/body system a chance to engage in the nutritional healing that has been covered.

ALIGN WITH NATURE'S DAILY RHYTHMS

For many, depression literally lowers energy in the body. It can make you feel sluggish, so all you feel you can do, or want to do, is lie around and retreat from the world. Other times it can cause anxiety and excitability, leaving you unable to focus or get proper rest and relaxation. People with depression tend to avoid participating in any activity that is not mandatory. They lose desire to do things they formerly enjoyed. They lose their appetites. They have troubling sleeping. Mentally, they're not alert. Their minds are running so slow that their thoughts seem fuzzy. Or they keep running and rerunning negative thoughts or conversations in their minds. They're easily distracted. The whole body can feel heavier. These signs of a brain/body imbalance signify that equilibrium needs to be restored.

Sleep

Your well-being is dependent on being able to function during your waking hours and being able to rest when you're asleep so your body may be restored. For this, you need deep, uninterrupted sleep at night—ideally for eight hours. As you sleep, your brain waves go through cycles. Without experiencing all of these, you just won't feel well or be as resilient.

Sleep research shows that it is important to practice good sleep "hygiene," which means:
- Avoid caffeine, nicotine, and other stimulants, such as sugar and spicy food within at least a couple of hours of going to bed.
- Power down your technology (computer/TV/smartphone) two hours before bed.
- Ensure complete darkness in the bedroom with "blackout" curtains or an eye mask.

- Maintain the same pattern of bedtime and rising every day, even on weekends.
- Do your best to rise with the light and to sleep with the darkness.
- Take nutritional supplements to replenish neurotransmitters involved with sleep (tryptophan or 5-HTP and melatonin).
- Stretch gently and meditate or read before lying down to fall asleep.
- Try aromatherapy: Diffuse lavender, Roman chamomile, and/or bergamot essential oil at bedtime.
- Maintain calm in the bedroom; always treat it as a sacred place.

Sunlight

The modern lifestyle overrides natural sleep cycles. We use electricity to power lights at night time when our biology would prefer us to settle down. By watching television and staring at the view screens on our computers and smartphones, we stimulate the pineal gland in the brain and this slows down the production of melatonin, a hormone our body secretes at night to help us fall asleep. This creates restlessness and insomnia at night when we should be settling down. The problem of sleeplessness is so pervasive today that in 2012, 60 million Americans filled prescriptions for sleeping pills.[1]

Seeing the natural light of the sun helps our brains and bodies to work better. Morning sunlight is most needed science shows, as it sets the internal clock for our bodies during the day.[2] In polar regions where there is little sunlight in the winter, doctors recognize a syndrome known as *seasonal affective disorder* (SAD), for which they prescribe daily exposure to a light box in the natural spectrum for thirty to sixty minutes.[3]

The fact that sunlight makes us happier and helps us stay mentally well is not disputed. Psychologist Michael Terman, author of *Reset Your Inner Clock*, claims this is not due to skin exposure but retinal exposure.[4] Contact to sunlight stimulates brain cells that impact our central nervous system and hormone regulation, ultimately affecting mood and mental focus.

There is a second reason to seek out sunshine: The body manufactures vitamin D when the skin is exposed to sunlight; and without it, we easily become deficient. It has been well documented that people with vitamin D deficiency tend to be depressed. Vitamin D deficiency has also been linked to diabetes 2, cancer, cardiovascular disease, and other conditions known to contribute to depression. It regulates immune response and reduces production of cytokines, which are responsible for inflammation. Also, it may increase the production of serotonin.[5]

Vitamin D is a fat-soluble vitamin. Although there are different sources, getting ive to fifteen minutes of exposure to sunlight daily on the face and hands is sufficient for the body to produce an optimal amount of vitamin D. Dark skin requires more time than fair skin for synthesis. Synthesis occurs when the skin reacts to UVB rays. Summer sunlight increases vitamin D twice as much as winter sunlight.[6]

Sources from food of vitamin D are: fungi and fish.

The beauty is that sunshine is free.

NATURAL EMOTIONS

There is nothing wrong with being sad from time to time. It is an appropriate response to loss or trauma. If you're grieving the death of a close friend or family member, or your house was swept away in a hurricane or mud slide, or you were told that you were being laid off from a job, you might expect to feel sad for a while. Such sadness is a signal of meaningful change.

When you're feeling blue and the mood becomes persistent, however, it is important to do something to keep yourself from spiraling further down. It's important to intervene to assist your body and mind in restoring equilibrium before you get trapped in a depressive state and, if at all possible, to avoid doing anything that reinforces your depression. It may take time before it is possible for you to make a mood switch from feeling angry, sad, forlorn, upset, or confused, to feeling remarkably upbeat: ecstatic, giddy, joyful, or exuberant. But . . . could you find a way to feel just a little bit better right away?

Think about it: If there was a simple thing you could do right now to feel a little better, what would that be? Stopping your reading right now to take a deep breath? Having a glass of water? Remembering something you're grateful for? Meditating for five minutes? Smiling across the room at your husband or wife? Petting your dog or cat? Stretching?

Have you ever noticed how your mood can shift suddenly when someone you love calls you? Or you hear a joke? Or a song comes on the radio that gets you humming? This remarkable potential lives inside the nervous system of each and every one of us.

Emotions are energy in motion. But sometimes we get stuck in a state of being that pains us: An emotion moves into the body like a demanding houseguest who has overstayed its welcome. If we resist feeling whatever it is we're feeling, we can actually cause ourselves more pain. But if we allow ourselves to take a minute to be with whatever we're feeling—no matter how unpleasant we find it or how ugly and inappropriate we believe it is—an emotion's grip on us weakens. Emotions are the body signaling us that something in us needs attention. These messages are an opportunity to practice self-nurturing, understanding, and compassion.

One of ten reasons that depression rates have been rising around the world is that we use the technology of the modern lifestyle to override the messages of our biology. We stay up past dark, don't move enough, and continuously stimulate our brains with rays of light from TVs and computer screens, so our bodies have begun to scream at us to get our attention. We tend to move fast, but if we slow down enough to "listen" with our senses to what we're feeling—and then respond with love, as we would to the needs of a small child in our care—then the natural healing response of our biology could restore our equilibrium.

If recently you suffered a meaningful loss or trauma, you may be grieving. Remember to give yourself time to process your feelings and adapt. Grief and trauma are stressful. If you're grieving or under stress, it is important to learn to recognize signs of your body's responses, such as having difficulty sleeping, being easily angered, feeling depressed, and having low energy. In search of comfort, some people are drawn to consume alcohol or other substances, or to overeat. These are false comforts, as they do not change the issue at its emotional roots.

Practice setting priorities for a while that give you room for emotional healing. Decide what must absolutely get done now or soon, and what can wait or even be put off forever; and learn to say no to taking on new tasks if they could heighten your sense of being overloaded. Make a point to note what you have accomplished at the end of the day, not what you have been unable to do. Although we've all been taught that it is appropriate to care for others, this is a good time to practice taking care of you. Being your number one priority may be necessary now.

Stay in touch with people who can provide you with emotional and other support. Ask for help from friends and family, and community or religious organizations, to reduce your stress due to work burdens or family issues, such as caring for a loved one who is ailing.

Avoid dwelling on your problems. If you can't do so on your own, seek help from a qualified mental health professional who can guide you. Do so if you are overwhelmed, feel you cannot cope, have suicidal thoughts, or are using drugs or alcohol to cope. Consider setting aside private time every day to immerse yourself in your feelings. Fall apart then, if you want to. Cry. Yell. Punch a pillow. The rest of the day, go about your regular activities as best as you can.

ESSENTIAL OILS FOR EMOTIONAL HEALING

Aromatherapy or topical application of essential oils may be therapeutic for managing difficult emotional states. Try these recipes for grief, emotional trauma, and anger.

Relief of Grief: Aromatic

Oil protocol: Combine equal parts of bergamot and lime oil; and if you have it available, add a small drop of jasmine or rose oil.

Application: Diffuse regularly.

Affirmation: Look into your eyes in the mirror (or imagine yourself standing in front of yourself looking into your eyes) and with compassion say out loud: *"It is okay to feel my feelings. I am safe and I can heal. I release the past and make room for beneficial change."*

For Relief of Emotional Trauma: Topical

Oil protocol: Combine sandalwood, bergamot, geranium, and lime oil; or blend frankincense, sandalwood, white fir, helichrysum, and rose oil.

Application: Apply over the lungs and chest and/or bottoms of your feet regularly, as needed.

Affirmation: Look into your eyes in the mirror (or imagine yourself standing in front of yourself looking into your eyes) and with compassion say out loud: *"I am healthy and well. I am whole and complete. I trust myself and I am safe. I embrace the future and I am free to be happy."*

Diminishing Anger: Aromatic

Oil protocol: Combine Roman chamomile, bergamot, and wild orange oil. Or use melissa oil only.

Application: Massage over your abdomen and inhale.

Affirmation: Look into your eyes in the mirror, or imagine yourself standing in front of yourself and looking into your own eyes with compassion, and say: *"I am learning to understand the root cause of my anger. I am making wise choices to sleep, heal, talk, and release my anger. I am happy with who I am. I am replacing anger with joy."*

Relief from Anger: Topical

Oil protocol: Combine bergamot, jasmine, and vetiver oil; or blend lavender and melissa oil.

Application: Apply to the sternum and bottoms of your feet.

Affirmation: Look into your eyes in the mirror (or imagine yourself standing in front of yourself looking into your eyes) and with compassion say out loud: *"I manage my emotions with ease and understanding. I am confident in my ability to remain calm and peaceful at all times."*

THE MOOD-LOWERING STRESS RESPONSE

The biggest problem with the modern lifestyle is that it is stressful. We put stress on ourselves through the thousands of small choices we make every day. Sometimes it seems like we've forgotten how to be human beings. Thinking that we are the masters of nature, instead of natural beings that are part of nature, it is easy to fall into a habit of overriding the body's various signals for sleep, for fresh air, for exercise, and in turn, for inactivity. Unfortunately, the effects of stress tend to build up over time, which means that taking practical steps to maintain our health and outlook is critical if we intend to reduce or prevent these effects.

When we tune back in after a stressful period, such as being on a deadline, studying for exams, or moving homes, or going through a divorce, we can observe whether we're bouncing back or feeling rundown. All the chemical reactions that take place in the body when we feel threatened, are normal, such as our heart rate and breathing rate increasing.

We are hard-wired to respond to threats and aggression in ways that will keep us safe: to flee or fight. Physiologically, the hypothalamus signals the adrenal glands to release a cascade of hormones, including adrenaline and cortisol, that are designed to transform us from mild-mannered Clark Kent into Superman. We become stronger, faster, and clearer thinking because our hearts beat faster, our blood pressure rises, and excitatory chemicals flood the brain. The transformation is made possible by repurposing energy and chemical resources from systems that are nonessential in the face of danger: digestion, reproduction, and growth.[7] That doesn't mean those systems are not necessary for our lives and our health! Just that Mother Nature wanted us to have a temporary boost so we wouldn't get crushed by an arch villain.

A lot is happening in the brain when we're feeling stressed. Norepinephrine is released to help us adapt to the challenge in front of us. What is maladaptive about this biological response pattern, however, is that our thoughts can make us react as if our very lives are at stake—even if they're not. Stress is subjective. Constant worry, overworking, boredom, loneliness, isolation, or feeling overwhelmed, powerless, or out of control, all put stress on us to different degrees. If our stress triggers go on for a long time without relief, such as they might if we were soldiering in a war or being bullied by a belligerent colleague in the workplace, we wear down. Sooner or later, chronic stress depletes our neurotransmitters, leading us to fatigue and possibly depression.

Interestingly, there is another response to stress that women are more prone to than men. It's called the *tend-and-befriend response*, which is caused by the release of the hormone oxytocin, which also functions as a neurotransmitter in the brain.[8] Oxytocin is more prevalent in the female of our species as it relates to bonding and trust, such as a mother and infant would feel. It is released when we hug or kiss a loved one, or have an orgasm. It connects us intimately. We'll look more closely at the emotional benefits of social bonding in the next chapter.

THE MOOD-ELEVATING RELAXATION RESPONSE

The autonomic nervous system (ANS), which regulates glands and organs in the body with no conscious involvement from us, has three parts to it. In the last chapter, we looked at the first of these subparts, the enteric nervous system, which controls actions in the GI tract. The second part of the nervous system, the part activated when we're under stress, is the *sympathetic nervous system*. The last part is the *parasympathetic nervous system,* which is responsible for actions related to rest/restoration, hunger/digestion, and sexual arousal/reproduction.[9]

The sympathetic and parasympathetic responses can be considered opposites. One stimulates us to act fast and tense up. The other stimulates us to slow down and relax. The relaxation response is mood elevating under ordinary circumstances, and immensely so when it provides relief from chronic stress. Our biology, if we're healthy and functioning optimally, can produce both responses when they're appropriate.

In 1975, Harvard Medical School associate professor, cardiologist, and founder of the Mind Body Medical Institute in Massachusetts, Herbert Benson, M.D., published the now-classic book *The Relaxation Response,* in which he explains how to elicit the parasympathetic nervous system and why it is so beneficial. Basically, the instructions are to sit or lie down (get comfortable), close your eyes, breathe through your nose, and count your exhalations ("one," "two," "three," and so on) for ten to twenty minutes. Give no thought to how well you're doing. Simply release your muscular tension. Be passive. Your biology will take care of its own needs. You cannot "force" relaxation. When you're done, take your time reengaging with your activities. Shift gears gradually, so as not to shock your system.[10]

What Benson is describing is known in some circles as mindfulness meditation. According to a reliable 2011 brain-imaging study, whose protocols were repeated in three different hospitals, two in the United States, one in Germany, mindfulness meditation produces measureable changes in regions in the brain associated with memory, learning, and emotions.[11]

If your depression is due to depletion from prolonged stress, you may need to engage in a resting mode frequently for a period to allow your body to thoroughly replenish itself. Spend a weekend purposefully walking slowly and napping whenever you're tired. Consider it a mini-retreat. Or actually go on retreat to a spa and get some massages. Play soothing music.

According to the American Institute of Stress, when eliciting the relaxation response:[12]
- Your metabolism decreases.
- Your levels of nitric oxide are increased, which is beneficial for the heart, immunity, and digestion.
- Your heart beats slower and your muscles relax.
- Your breathing becomes slower.
- Your blood pressure decreases.

AROMATHERAPY TO LIFT YOUR SPIRITS

The scents of lavender and vanilla decrease anxiety and improve symptoms of depression and insomnia.

MINDFULNESS: YOGA, TAI CHI, AND CONTROLLED BREATHING

In 1997, neuroscientist and pharmacologist Candace B. Pert, Ph.D., who discovered the opiate receptor, the binding site in the brain for endorphins, our feel-good neurotransmitters, wrote a letter to *Time* magazine. Her pioneering research led to the development of modern antidepressant drugs, such as Prozac. That letter reads:

> *"I am alarmed at the monster that Johns Hopkins neuroscientist Solomon Snyder and I created when we discovered the simple binding assay for drug receptors 25 years ago. . . . The public is being misinformed about the precision of these selective serotonin-uptake inhibitors when the medical profession oversimplifies their action in the brain and ignores the body as if it exists merely to carry the head around! In short, these molecules of emotion regulate every aspect of our physiology. A new paradigm has evolved, with implications that life-style changes such as diet and exercise can offer profound, safe and natural mood elevation."*[13]

Considering the potential side effects of antidepressant medication, lifestyle modification should come first. Some studies suggest that forms of exercise which incorporate awareness and movement, such as yoga and tai chi, are particularly beneficial for overcoming depression.[14]

Yoga

How does it work as a mood elevator? A study in the *Journal of Alternative and Complementary Medicine* found that yoga increased the level of GABA in people's brains.[15] Low levels are connected with anxiety and depression. GABA has a calming influence on us. Researchers from Duke University analyzed the results of 124 trials and found a clear benefit for people suffering from depression.[16]

Stretching

Researchers studied eighty young adults diagnosed with mild to moderate depression for twelve weeks to determine what forms of exercise brought relief. The published results reveal that depressive symptoms were reduced:[17]
- Fifty percent for those who did thirty minutes of high-intensity, aerobic exercise three to five times a week.
- Thirty percent for those who did low-intensity exercise three to five times a week.
- Twenty-nine percent for those who did stretching fifteen to twenty minutes per day.

Tai Chi

A survey of 529 Japanese tai chi practitioners was conducted, assessing them by different measures related to quantity, quality, and years of practice. Researchers concluded: "This study has demonstrated that long-term tai chi training is independently related to a lower prevalence of depressive symptoms. These results suggest that long-term tai chi training may have a beneficial effect on the prevention of depressive symptoms."[18]

Controlled Breathing

In their article, "The Science of Breathing," University of Arizona researchers Sarah Novotny and Len Kravitz, Ph.D., assert, "How we breathe can change our psychophysiological state. One therapeutic goal of yoga is that it may reduce or alleviate some of the chronic negative effects of stress. This stress relief is one reason that breathing, or pranayama, as it is called in yoga, is very central to yoga practices."[19]

Stress is the brain's response to positive or negative demands. It can be invigorating, like riding a rollercoaster, getting married, going on a first date, or winning a competition. It can be lifesaving, if you are running from an angry bull in Pamplona, Spain, or just fell overboard on a cruise ship. No matter what the demand is the pulse quickens, we breathe faster, our muscles get tense, and brain activity increases. Other physiological functions are suppressed for the duration, which is why stress lowers our immunity to colds and flu. Stress uses up our resources.

Controlled breathing reverses the stress response. Sudarshan kriya yoga (SKY), a type of controlled breathing that has roots in traditional yoga, shows great promise in providing relief for depression. The program involves several types of cyclical breathing patterns, ranging from slow and calming to rapid and stimulating. In a study of people hospitalized for depression who used SKY for four weeks, 67 percent achieved remission versus 73 percent who took a drug and 93 percent of those who underwent electroconvulsive therapy.[20]

Breathing to Relieve Depression

When we are feeling down in the dumps, the following practice can help you regulate your ANS through breathing.

Begin by finding a comfortable place to sit down or lie down.

Then, relax and expand the body with parasympathetic breathing, creating space for energy to flow. Focus on bringing the breath in through the nose and moving it down into the lower abdomen; and then releasing a long, sighing exhale through the mouth. Exhales should be much slower than inhales. Aim for a two-to-one or a three-to-one ratio.

Once the body is relaxed and your musculature has expanded, move on to a stimulating breathing technique. In states of low arousal, such as depression, it is important to arouse your nervous system to acquire a sense of aliveness and heightened energy.

Sympathetic breathing techniques involve breathing into the upper chest, all the way up to the upper ribs and collar bones. Imagine you are panting, but through your nose, almost like a runner calling up energy for her muscles. In this type of quicker breathing, the inhalation should be emphasized.

Alternate one minute of slow breathing, followed by one minute of quick breathing. Repeat the alternation three times. Then end with a few minutes of regular, uncontrolled breathing. Just rest and let your body restore its own balance.

Eucalyptus essential oil is helpful for breathing. It would be useful to apply it topically when conducting any breathing exercise.

VIGOROUS EXERCISE

Almost any type of strenuous physical activity, from running, rowing, and swimming to salsa dancing is capable of stimulating the brain to release endorphins in the brain and body. Endorphin production doesn't always happen. But it is immensely pleasurable when it does. Similar to morphine, endorphin can bring about both pain relief and euphoria. Long distance runners have become so familiar with this safe, naturally occurring phenomenon that it is now known as the *runner's high*.[21]

To trigger this biological response requires at least 20–30 minutes or longer of sustained movement at a moderate intensity—below the threshold of fatigue. Apparently it needs to be rhythmic and predictable (which is why running is such a great gateway for this phenomenon—and so is salsa dancing). Duration matters. As the body compensates for the challenge of the increased demand for oxygen and energy, the heart rate goes up and blood flow increases, the joints become lubricated with synovial fluid, and the mind becomes calmer and clearer. Occasional bursts of speed or intensity in the midst of your workout can persuade the body it has to perform at an even higher level.[22] With its innate intelligence, it releases endorphins to energize you and help you keep going, as our ancient ancestors needed to do to hunt animals on foot they intended to eat. Once endorphins are circulating in the bloodstream, you feel invigorated, like you could go on forever.

Different types of athletes have been studied under various conditions. According to researchers, having company or listening to up tempo music can boost the euphoric effect.[23] Because hormones are replenished after a good night's sleep, some suggest that morning exercise increases the likelihood of having this response.[24]

If you're not persuaded to exercise yet, consider the following bit of news about changing the structure of the brain! James S. Gordon, M.D., one of the world's most renowned experts in mind-body medicine, has said:

> *"What we're finding in the research on physical exercise is that exercise is at least as good as antidepressants for helping people who are depressed . . . Exercise can increase the number of cells in your brain, in the region*

of the brain called the hippocampus. These studies were first done on animals, and they're very important because sometimes in depression, there are fewer of those cells in the hippocampus. But you can actually change your brain with exercise. So it's got to be part of everybody's treatment, everybody's plan."[25]

CHANGE YOUR POSTURE

Did you know that just shifting your posture can change your mood and state of mind? It makes a lot of sense once you start thinking about the brain's need for oxygen and how impactful rhythmic, controlled breathing is. Depressed people tend to hunch forward and keep their heads low. This compresses the rib cage and makes the diaphragm cave in. Thus, it's hard for them to take in oxygen and the body reacts by slowing down to decrease the demand for oxygen.[26]

What's the remedy? Since the body is very intelligent, if you throw your shoulders back, lift your head, expand your rib cage, and take some good, strong, deep breaths in, your ANS will be stimulated and your will mood lift!

Try it for yourself. Breathing mechanics are such that we can dictate to our bodies how to feel. If you're feeling hyper-aroused, you have the power to slow yourself down. If you're feeling hypo-aroused, you can also speed yourself up.

ESTABLISHING A FIELD OF POSITIVE ENERGY AROUND YOU

Declare that it is your intention to be happy from now on.

Apply an essential oil: Combine wild orange and peppermint and diffuse.

Say an affirmation: *"I am extraordinarily positive and I maintain healthy boundaries. Everyone around me is happy, helpful, and delightful. Everyone around me supports me in creating positive energy."*

Recipe for a Natural Mood-Enhancing Lifestyle

- Fresh air, as much as possible
- Sunlight, 15 minutes in the morning on face and hands
- Green environment, an everyday connection with nature
- Vigorous exercise, 30 minutes per day
- Relaxation/stretching, 20 minutes per day
- Meditation, 15 minutes, morning and night
- Aromatherapy with essential oils, as needed
- Sleep, 8 hours per night
- Get proper health care for existing or new health problems

Mother Nature's Answer 3

Happy Relationships

There is compelling evidence that we are happier and more resilient when we are connected to other people. Human beings are social creatures. We are wired to function best through cooperation and human connection. Historically, our ancestors needed one another to build cultures and civilizations to support the growth of human kind. The very survival of our species depends upon our ability to work well with others, to love, to forgive, to alter the way we think, and to negotiate and clean up problems in our relationships. When we can't do these things, we threaten our social structure from the very minutest connections to the largest cultural networks.

For the sake of happiness, two kinds of relationships matter: the relationship with self and the relationship with anyone inside the circle of family/trust—let's call it the *tribe*—including close friends and domestic animals. In part, we define our identities through our social bonds: through those who know us and love us, and those whom we want to support and demonstrate allegiance to. When our tribal relationships are healthy, they promote happiness. Although tremendously rewarding at times, family relationships have multiple layers of meaning associated with them and they can be intensely challenging, too.

The person we assign ourselves to be is the self we create through our constant interaction inside our minds: not only do we interact with a voice we "hear" inside our heads (our thoughts), but we have feelings about the qualities and capabilities we possess, to which we assign individual worth. Essentially, who we are gets expressed through the lens of our own personal judgments, values, and inner beliefs. How we relate to our bodies, beliefs, thoughts, feelings, and desires can be complicated by depression—but sometimes depression is a valuable message that it is time to focus on healing. Discomfort can lead to awareness, which gives us an opportunity to heal, set wellness goals, and make better choices.

Due to advances in brain imaging, we now know that we are growing new neural networks our entire lives: We are literally *changing our minds*. We have an extraordinary capacity for learning and adaptation. And while it can and does happen naturally, biological transformation is a process that also, fortunately, can be cultivated on purpose.

Emotions are byproducts of our biology.

WE ARE NATURALLY EMOTIONAL BEINGS

In a speech given in 1938, psychologist Carl Gustav Jung, whose work has influenced psychiatry, religion, and literature for more than seventy years, said, "Emotion is the chief source of all becoming-conscious."[1] Feelings are amazing, complex messengers that can teach us about ourselves. When and how they are felt is unique to each individual's experience, yet every emotion is available to all of us. Fear, anger, sadness, frustration, resentment, terror, love, joy, peace, forgiveness, gratitude, and happiness are universally recognized. We all experience these same emotions to some degree throughout our lives, and we must learn to manage them.

How we interpret and regulate our emotions is critical to leading a happy life. In his classic 1995 book, *Emotional Intelligence*, psychologist and journalist Daniel Goleman explores the dimensions of EI, and offers evidence for why our ability to identify, use, understand, and manage our emotions is at least as important as our IQ.

In reporting on the cost of emotional illiteracy, Goleman states: "In navigating our lives, it is our fears and envies, our rages and depressions, our worries and anxieties that steer us day to day. Even the most academically brilliant among us are vulnerable to being undone by unruly emotions. The price we pay for emotional illiteracy is in failed marriages and troubled families, in stunted social and work lives, in deteriorating physical health and mental anguish and, as a society, in tragedies such as killings." Goleman says the best remedy for our emotional shortcomings is prevention: doing what we can to increase our emotional intelligence.[2]

According to psychologists from Yale University and the University of New Hampshire, emotional intelligence encompasses the following five characteristics and abilities.[3]
- **Self-awareness:** knowing your emotions, recognizing feelings as they occur, and discriminating between them.
- **Self-regulation:** handling feelings so they are relevant to the current situation and reacting appropriately. Essentially, monitoring, evaluating, and sometimes acting to change a mood.
- **Self-motivation:** using your emotions to direct yourself toward a goal, despite self-doubt, inertia, and impulsiveness.
- **Empathy:** recognizing feelings in others by being attuned to verbal and nonverbal cues.
- **Social skill:** managing relationships by handling interpersonal interaction, resolving conflicts, and negotiating.

The EI skill set is the one to draw upon any time you feel blue. When it comes to regulating moods by taking action, you can either do more of the things you like and which make you feel happier (mood maintenance), or do less of the things you don't like and which make you feel worse (mood repair). The ideal scenario is to intercede before your emotions spiral down into the low-energy state of depression.

A third option is to take no action, but rather to witness our emotions. Often awareness itself is enough for equilibrium to be spontaneously restored.

Let's begin with a look at ways to increase emotional awareness.

SPONTANEOUS HEALING THROUGH EMOTIONAL AWARENESS

For some people, depression is a result of suppressing painful memories, thoughts, and feelings. So much energy is put into burying memory of a traumatic event or an emotion, such as anger or shame, that insufficient life force remains for living. All feelings become suppressed, including positive feelings. Life can be harsh, but if pain is turned inward and buried, rather than processed and released, the nervous system shuts down around that emotional information.

When we begin to allow emotions and trauma to resurface, it can feel like we're being flooded and we can get overwhelmed. If this happens to you, and you're in need of support, please go and talk to somebody: a minister, a therapist, a trusted friend. Be gentle and go slowly if you're processing strong memories. Allow yourself plenty of time to grieve whatever comes up. Join a support group if it's appropriate to your situation. For example: a grief recovery group.

As suppression ends, you may find that you have a wild amount of energy running through your system. Be sure to nurture yourself with healthy lifestyle habits, such as exercise, that release tension. When things seem intense and exhausting, take a break: Go see a funny movie, work out at the gym, or hang out with a friend and do something silly. Take. A. Break.

Two techniques have been shown by research studies to help bring the light of awareness to issues that underlie depression. In using these, you may find that your mood lifts.

Therapeutic Writing and Journaling

In a study conducted at Southern Methodist University, social psychologist James W. Pennebaker found that writing about upsetting emotional experiences was therapeutic: significant physical and mental health improvements were initiated, including a reduction of distress.[4] The outcome was the same for people of different ages, races, and genders, "from honor students to maximum-security prisoners," writing about everything from lost love, to sexual abuse, and "tragic failure." Many of the subjects reported crying as they disclosed their pain on paper.[5]

Adapted from Pennebaker, the instructions for how this technique works are simple. For three to five days in a row, for approximately twenty minutes write about your deepest thoughts and feelings as related to an extremely important emotional issue that has affected your life. Let go and explore. Give no thought to grammar, spelling, or cognitive coherence. This writing is intended for you alone to read. You may tie your thoughts and feelings to your relationships or to your past, present, or future. Feel free to write about the same issue or a different issue every day. The important thing is to write for the entire duration of the day's writing session.

Another technique you can try is simply keeping a journal. Keeping track of the thoughts that plague us and are connected to our unhappiness can begin to raise our awareness. After a period, go back and reread your old journal entries. Look for themes. See if there are any clues that can help you regulate your emotions better.

Meditation

On his blog, Deepak Chopra writes: "Meditation trains your mind to become aware of the silent witness within you that is independent of the universe you are observing. This core self is not a philosophical or theological concept; it is an experience of your authentic existence. With an established sense of the silent witness, it will be easier to not become identified with the darkness of your depressed days."[6] When we access this witnessing ability it gives us chance to step back. This can bring relief—even if only temporary relief—from a painful reality.

Try a simple, non-demanding meditation that lasts five minutes. The steps are few.
1. Sit comfortably and close your eyes. Be still.
2. Breathe naturally without changing anything.
3. Begin paying attention to the sensations of your breath in your body.
4. If you notice any tension or holding simply let it go.
5. Stay with your breath as it enters and leaves your body.

You can increase the amount of time you spend meditating whenever you want. Even a few minutes of meditating like this are soothing to the nervous system. Meditating a couple of times a day may help you begin to overcome painful sensations and feelings you've stored in your body. As your awareness rises, you'll soon find ways to maintain your positive mood and avoid tension.

In a different article, the Chopra Center newsletter rightly asserts, "The emotional effects of sitting quieting and going within are profound. The deep state of rest produced by meditation triggers the brain to release neurotransmitters, including dopamine, serotonin, oxytocin, and endorphins."[7]

WHAT ARE YOU THINKING? MAKE IT ADVANTAGEOUS

Today, we know that the instant a thought occurs, your hypothalamus—a "control center" at the base of your brain—turns that thought into hundreds of neuropeptides, each one associated with the dominant emotion of the corresponding thought. Those neuropeptides representing your thoughts are actual molecules being transmitted throughout your mind and body. If you feel depressed or joyful, it is a whole-body experience largely caused by these tiny messengers.[8]

Candace Pert, Ph.D., a neuroscientist and pharmacologist who pioneered much of the early work in mind-body medicine, found that neuropeptides are carried through the bloodstream and transmitted from one neuron to another. Each neuropeptide interlocks with a special receptor on the receiving neuron's membrane, just like a key fitting into a keyhole. The amino acids in each neuropeptide are then absorbed by your cells, causing your thoughts to become an actual, tangible part of the cells in your body![9]

How those cells change over time depends on the nature of your thinking.

According to Dr. Pert's research, the body's cells develop more and more specialized receptors for the neuropeptides to which they are most exposed. In fact, cells will even begin to crave these neuropeptides and ask the hypothalamus to produce them.[10] Over time, your cells thus wind up causing you to fulfill an emotional prophecy that affects your health and mood.

In other words, you get what you think about, whether you like it or not.

Understanding the power of thoughts and beginning to regulate them is critical to permanently solving psychological and physical conditions.

Let's compare the process of your thoughts forming chemical reactions to the process of a news agency, such as Associated Press, writing and distributing the daily news publication. Every day, writers and editors produce articles based on their research and perceptions of the latest information available in our world. The articles are then printed in a newspaper or posted on a website. Similarly, you have the opportunity every day to write your own news (aka choose your own thoughts) based on your perceptions of the happenings in your world. This news (your thoughts) is published in the form of neuropeptides that get delivered to the cells within your body. Just as world news becomes the reality of the world we live in when we act on it, so do your thoughts create your own reality, which can include your health and well-being.

Every day, every moment, your cells are waiting for more information from you: the latest news. When it comes, they respond accordingly. When day in and day out you "deliver" the same morning news (provide the same thoughts) to your body, you establish specific neurological pathways that alter your biochemistry. This is how habitual thinking patterns are created and maintained.

Habitual thought patterns create matching body chemistry. Until different news is presented to your body on a regular basis and overrides the original message, your neuropeptides will follow the same pathways back to your original messaging or thinking.

In recent years, it has become popular increasingly to use positive affirmations to guide thoughts. This technique can be tremendously effective. There are also programs in the marketplace that employ subliminal means to speak to the unconscious mind, helping listeners to re-pattern their thoughts at the deepest levels. Forms of hypnosis, acupuncture, meditation, eye-movement therapy, tapping techniques, body awareness therapy, emotional processing, energy work, and massage are being implemented and used to help us change our instincts and beliefs. Try some, and see what happens for you.

Committing to re-patterning your thoughts on your own can be a powerful way to make changes to your body chemistry. This process is important—maybe even critical—to helping you create a happy and healthy life. It is best not to say affirmations when you are in bad space or angry. Rather focus on positive change and encouraging goals.

It doesn't always feel like it, but we do have the ability to stop a thought in its tracks and replace it with a better thought. Even though it may feel artificial at first, when you do this repeatedly, it becomes easier. For instance, a woman who was often triggered to feel victimized when she was asked to work overtime caught herself muttering under her breath, "Just shoot me and put me out of my misery." Witnessing this gave her a bit of control. She decided to substitute a positive thought that she liked better: "Just make me happy!"

And guess what? It really did.

After using "I am becoming happy" and "I am happy now" as affirmations, she discovered that a lot of her depressed feelings had been related to feeling powerless. Once she changed the tone of her thoughts, she felt empowered to make other changes.

BELIEFS

Like computers with complex processing systems, the body contains all the facets of an individual's perceptions. Your personal body computer may change daily as new information is put in and outdated information is replaced by new understanding. Alternatively, your personal body computer may rarely change: running and re-running old data over and over again. If you make decisions about others and yourself and lock these perceptions into your body/mind computer (usually by repetition), your system begins to filter your experiences through the beliefs and feelings you have stored.

Let's take a look at Sam. As a child of delinquent parents, his mind/body was fed constant cues that led him to feel unworthy and undeserving. Over time, Sam began to see all circumstances through a tainted lens. Even after he was no longer surrounded by people who treated him poorly or with reckless abandon, Sam began blocking out other views of reality that existed simultaneously. Although he saw every experience as validation of his worthlessness, all the while many of his experiences could be seen by others to be opposite to his perception.

Here's another, more visual example of this concept. When you buy a new car, you become instantly familiar with that car's model and color. In fact, from that point on you notice cars like yours whenever you are driving. In the past, you may not have really paid attention to navy blue Honda Pilots. But now you seem to notice every single one on the road. Fast forward ten years or more down the road, and it's likely you're still noticing all the navy blue Honda Pilots on the road, even if you sold yours by then.

So it is with each of us in our lives. When we have experiences that lead us to make decisions about our lives or ourselves, we unconsciously go out into the world and notice all other experiences that validate what we believe to be true. Certainly there were just as many red Honda Pilots driving around all those years; but somehow you noticed only the blue ones.

This is also the way the brain processes emotions and experiences. When the brain makes a decision about an experience or an emotion, it often holds on to that perception and will attempt to recreate similar circumstances or feelings to validate those beliefs. Someone like Sam may expect that everyone abandons those they love. He may not recognize that healthy relationships do exist. Abandonment—his navy blue Honda Pilot—is all he sees, even if he parks right next to a shiny red minivan every day at work.

Now imagine if "navy blue" was synonymous with "guilt" or "sadness." What if all your perceptions of life were being colored by your memories of childhood abuse, so that all you saw in your daily interactions and experiences were more occasions of abuse? Wouldn't you feel worse?

Fortunately, Sam doesn't have to be stuck in a rut. He can start to notice the other cars on the road, to recognize that other paths exist, and that many, many relationships can move forward without any fear of abandonment. All he needs to do is start feeding his body and mind new information and changing his perceptions.

This is true for each of us as well, no matter what we've been though. With self-exploration, take some time to discover the truth behind your beliefs, to look at the reality you have created and see if that reality might be skewed by your perceptions. If it is, start feeding your mind new information. Reshape your reality and, in turn, you can reshape your vitality.

IMPERFECTION IS PERFECT FOR MOTHER NATURE

For perfectionists, anything they decide to do that lies outside their comfort zone can seem like a one-way ticket to unhappiness, as negative emotions and self-critical thoughts can take them over. If this happens frequently, this pattern may become so painful that they try to medicate it with alcohol or food . . . and sometimes it results in addiction, leading to depression. The definition of a perfectionist is someone who strives for flawlessness and high achievement, but does not account for the stages of learning that go into mastery of their skills.

What gets a perfectionist into trouble is turning the desire to achieve a high standard into a focus on avoiding failure. This type of negative focus drags perfectionists into an emotional puddle of misery. Trying to avoid failure is counterproductive in a world where we often learn the most from the mistakes we make while trying to find a solution that works!

Perfectionists become perfectionists because they learned early in life that they could only gain the approval and love of meaningful people through accomplishment. Consequently, the self-esteem of perfectionists is based primarily on external standards and expectations. This leaves them vulnerable and sensitive to the opinions of those around them.

We human beings are so concerned about being loved that on a subconscious level we thirst for love as much as we do for food and water. In order to protect themselves from criticism or ridicule, and be "worthy of love," perfectionists work hard to be all things for all people—to the point of exhaustion. If and when they fail to gain the approval of others, perfectionists can end up being miserable, fatigued, depleted, and unresilient until they process negative emotions that have arisen, such as fear, sadness, guilt, shame, and anger.

Perfectionists typically don't know who they are. They are commonly lost in their own thoughts and feelings, always living in a world of "shoulds" that are dictated by the opinions of others. They live with guilt, compliance, defiance, and shame. They have little or no self-worth. They cannot take a compliment. Even when others in their lives provide them with positive feedback, they are not satisfied! They don't know how to identify personal satisfaction. Negative feedback sends them into a downward spiral of depression.

For perfectionists, the following issues crop up regularly: fear of failure, fear of making mistakes, fear of disapproval, all-or-nothing thinking (which leads perfectionists to be out-of-balance and lose prospective), an overemphasis on "shoulds," believing that others are more easily successful than them, and a lot of guilt and judgment. Until and unless healing occurs, and they develop self-esteem, self-approval cannot provide the validation they desire.

Interestingly, there is a healthy side to perfectionism. In fact, psychologists now group perfectionism into two categories: *adaptive* (healthy) perfectionism and *maladaptive* (unhealthy) perfectionism.[11] The distinction is that healthy perfectionists aren't afraid of failure. They set high standards and remain self-confident, even if they can't seem to achieve their desired outcomes. Maladaptive perfectionists live in a world where under the same conditions they beat themselves up—never feeling good enough and rarely feeling happy with accomplishments.

If you believe that perfectionism is making you miserable, set aside some time for self-reflection and reformulating your thought patterns. To break out of your pattern of painful and paralyzing self-criticism and let go of the "shoulds" that have defined you to date, get comfortable and then connect with your inner thoughts, feelings, and desires. Apply bergamot, lavender, wild orange, eucalyptus, lime, rosemary, or frankincense oil on your chest and inhale while focusing on the statement: *"I am comfortable with choosing to feel good all of the time."*

In *Conversations with Myself*, Nobel Peace Prize-winner Nelson Mandela writes: "In judging our progress as individuals, we tend to concentrate on external factors such as one's social position, influence and popularity, wealth and standard of education. These are, of course, important in measuring one's success in material matters and it is perfectly understandable if many people exert themselves mainly to achieve all these. But internal factors may be even more crucial in assessing one's development as a human being. Honesty, sincerity, simplicity, humility, pure generosity, absence of vanity, readiness to serve others—qualities which are within easy reach of every soul—are the foundation of one's spiritual life."[12]

SOCIAL INTELLIGENCE AND BRAIN FUNCTION

Do you sometimes feel drained when you're in an environment with extraordinarily negative people? It's possible that what you're feeling may be more than just an emotional response; their negativity may be affecting your health. Conversely, think of how great you feel when you are with someone who always focuses on the positive, seeks the silver lining in every situation, tries to do good, wants to be supportive, and fills your mind with uplifting thoughts.

During a study on meditation years ago, a group of doctors working with mind/body expert Deepak Chopra verified that meditation increases serotonin levels in the brain.[13] They also realized that those who were not participating in the meditations but were involved with the study on a regular basis also had experienced an increase of serotonin in the brain. In other words, the study itself was spreading happy feelings. The researchers concluded that positive attitudes can physiologically benefit those with whom we associate on a regular basis.[14]

Our moods have a powerful impact on the people around us. Just think about it: How easy is it for one grumpy family member to ruin the environment of a home? Or for an enraged or irritable employee to destroy the morale of an entire office? It's a truism that one bad apple has the potential to spoil the entire barrel. That's why each of us has a responsibility to choose happiness, not just for our personal benefit, but for everyone's benefit.

Selfish people are generally very unhappy. Usually selfishness stems from a sense of deprivation and fear that personal needs are not going to be met. Even if you think selfishness helps you feel fulfilled, it turns out that those who forget their troubles through service to others find happiness. A 1992 study of altruistic behavior found that self-esteem and a sense of well-being increased by as much as 24 percent for those who served.[15] In fact, it was the simple acts of kindness that produced the reward—generous actions, like holding the door open for others, thanking the mail carrier or doorman, and helping an elderly person carry groceries.[16]

Really, it only takes a small shift in attitude to produce positive results in our lives.

When you feel grumpy, sad, or just plain miserable, remember your personal responsibility to be happy, and begin to serve others by healing your grumpy mood. Fulfill your responsibility by turning your negative tone into a positive influence.

That may seem easier said than done, of course. And it is. When you are emotionally overloaded and can't muster up the ability to put a smile on your face, forcing or pretending you've had an instant change of mood isn't realistic. So here are a few tips for clearing the dark cloud that's hanging over your head and bringing in powerful light.

- Visualize blowing all your frustrations, fears, anger, or whatever else you're feeling that's negative into an imaginary balloon. Watch inside your mind as this balloon lifts up high into the sky and eventually explodes in the light of the sun.
- Listen to beautiful, uplifting music.
- Go for a walk in nature.
- As the lyrics of the song "My Favorite Things," sung by Julie Andrews in *The Sound of Music*, suggest, make a list of your favorite things when you're feeling bad. Be sure to include all that you're grateful for.

OUR NEED FOR HUMAN CONNECTION

When it comes to depression, having supportive, intimate relationships can make a big difference. You see, attachment or belonging is an innate biological need.

In anthropologist Ashley Montagu's groundbreaking 1971 book, *Touching*, which opened people's eyes to the phenomenon, he describes the importance of tactile interaction to psychological well-being and explains how touching the skin can boost our immune function.[17] Infants who are not touched enough can "fail to thrive." And so can adults.

Touch is something everyone needs to be happy. So when you need an emotional lift, make a point to give and receive hugs, to hold hands walking down the street, to spoon your spouse in bed, to pet an animal, or to get a massage. Regular physical contact—especially skin-to-skin contact—is decidedly beneficial.

Results of a 2006 study funded by the Hope for Depression Research Foundation, which involved fMRI brain imaging, suggested that adults who had insecure attachment to their mothers in the first years of their lives are more prone to anxiety, depression, and personality disorders later in life.[18] Researchers looking for ways to measure propensity for depression, found that the area that lights up on diagnostic tests when people look at photographs of their mothers is the same one associated with conflict and social interactions.[19]

When you look at a photograph of your own mother, what emotions does it elicit?

If you had a traumatic childhood, you will likely need to do some healing work on issues related to your mother and other significant caregivers who should have protected you and shown you love. Sadness promotes sad thought patterns, so you may want to turn to cognitive therapy if you have internalized a feeling of not being worthy of love and care. Energy therapy, such as Reiki or emotional freedom technique (EFT), may also be helpful.

Interestingly, oxytocin, the hormone that bonds mothers to newborn babies when they nurse, serves as a neurotransmitter in the brain for both genders (men, too), where it aids in social recognition. Oxytocin is released by the pituitary gland whenever we hug, touch, or orgasm during lovemaking.[20] Animal studies designed to test oxytocin's impact on the brain have revealed that not only does it affect risk aversion, it also decreases the fear response.[21]

Perhaps oxytocin's role in ensuring the biological imperative of mothers to protect vulnerable youngsters explains why the fight-or-flight response is often modulated in women by an inhibitory reflex that researchers have deemed the *tend-and-befriend response*. For men and women alike, the key reaction to a threat is the release of adrenal hormones. But instead of fleeing, women draw strength from forming alliances and bonding with other women and with the men who are their partners in life. These social connections relax women and decrease their fear, so that they can stay put for their children instead of being mobilized to run away. Men are less likely than women to have high levels of oxytocin, so they bond differently. And when stressed, men tend to withdraw or become aggressive, rather than seeking social support.[22]

HEALING YOUR FAMILY PATTERNS

Many of the patterns of behavior that we learn in the home thrive for generations in our families before anyone realizes there's another way to do things. Some of these patterns are destructive and damaging. Others are simply less effective ways of functioning.

Consider this funny example. One day, a newly married woman was getting ready to put a ham in the oven for her first

Sunday dinner at home with her new husband and her in-laws. Her husband watched with questioning eyes as she pulled the ham out of the refrigerator to prepare it and immediately cut off two inches from both ends. She seasoned the meat plopped it in the pan, moved it to the oven, and then unceremoniously threw away the ends of the ham! It took a little courage for the man to question his wife as she readied the rest of the meal, but he finally spurted out, "Why on Earth did you throw away those perfectly good ends of the ham?"

Baffled, the wife responded, "Well, isn't that the way you're supposed to cook a ham?" After some discussion with her husband, the wife decided to call her mother to get proof that this, indeed, was the proper way to cook a ham. "Mom," she said, as she handed her husband the phone in exasperation, "will you please explain to Joe why it's important to cut off the ends of the ham." Her mom somewhat sheepishly replied that she didn't actually know the reason; she'd just watched her own mother do it that way for years. This prompted a call to Grandma . . . and a few good laughs a few weeks later after the proverbial smoke of the argument had cleared. Grandma's response? "Well, I only had this tiny pan. The ham your grandfather brought home from the butcher never fit, so I just cut off the ends. Maybe I should have bought a bigger pan."

Take a moment and think about the story of the ham. The consequences of following this precedent without question were small in this case. But what if the precedent isn't in how you cook a ham, but how you react to a child who shatters a plate or a spouse who doesn't do exactly what you ask? If you're the first in a family line to want to break an ineffective or unhealthy pattern of thought or emotion, changing it may seem more difficult than moving a mountain. But it's not. It just takes time, work, and more time. It is possible—and worth it.

How do we transform depressive beliefs that have been ingrained for generations of time? In my book *Healing Your Family History*, I teach a five-step process, which can be applied to changing any pattern of thought or negative habit. In brief, this process involves:
1. Identifying your family's beliefs and traditions,
2. Overcoming judgments and fears,
3. Pushing out of your comfort zone and making fresh choices,
4. Finding the treasure that the family pattern masked, and
5. Forging a bond with your spirit, the part of you that knows your worth.

Certainly, we are vulnerable to our families when we are born. Not only are our little, delicate bodies dependent on others for the basics of life—food, safety, and shelter—we also look to our parents and other family members, and even our culture, for our sense of value and purpose. Early on, our parents, teachers, leaders, and communities play a huge role in dictating who we are and what we will become. Because we are young and impressionable, we tend to absorb their verbal and nonverbal scripts for us as the basis of our way of thinking about ourselves, and then we create our lives to match—that is, unless we become enlightened.

Our perceptions of ourselves are often based on the opinions, thoughts, and words of others. It's common that when a mother believes her child is bound for success and is beautiful and gracious, the child grows up to be successful, and to radiate beauty and graciousness. By contrast, if a mother believes that her child is a troublemaker, foolish, selfish, or worthless, it's likely that the child will manifest the negative script by thinking and behaving accordingly. Because our feelings about ourselves shape our lives, understanding these scripts and roles we're assigned by others, and their mood-diminishing effects on us, is crucial. Furthermore, understanding and rewriting the unhealthy scripts we project on others is also crucial because in freeing people from playing those roles we also free ourselves and have better relationships.

The good news is that you can alter your life by changing the scripts—not only the ones given to you, but the ones you give to others. You don't have to subordinate your power to the opinions of others, and you can teach your loved ones that they don't have to either. As the great runner, author, and philosopher George Sheehan said, "Success means having the courage, the determination, and the will to become the person you believe you were meant to be."[23]

How do you change the scripts and help yourself think differently? First, you need to know what you want, who you really are, and what you desire to become. You need a vision of your highest and best self, and you need a dream. Then you must anchor yourself in this purpose.

Gregg Braden tells a powerful story in his book *The Divine Matrix*. He explains how invincible we are when we fully focus ourselves on a meaningful dream. Years ago he was enrolled in a martial arts class. One day he showed up for class and the teacher announced a change in the agenda. The teacher told the group (some of his finest students) that he wanted them to knock him over. He took a minute to anchor himself to the ground. Assuming the task was easy, a few students tried to shove him. When they realized he wasn't budging, the whole group ganged up on one side to knock him over. Still, the teacher remained stable and strong. Why? Later the teacher explained that before the exercise, he had anchored himself deep within his consciousness by visualizing that he was sitting between mountains and that he was firmly chained to his position. His perceived reality became so strong in his mind that it outweighed the laws of physics. In other words, his dream (or vision) was so solid no one could topple him.[24]

When your thoughts, beliefs, and biochemistry support you in being solidly who you are, you become able to withstand the judgments, criticism, attacks, and hurtful projections of others regardless of your family history. Likewise, when you are solid in your dreams, you can overcome all odds and achieve them.

All of our families pass along traditions. Some of these traditions promote success, encourage love, and serve and heal those who choose to participate in them. Others can be both negative and positive. Some family traditions come without any good. Families who pass along dark abuse and hate, for instance, pass along patterns of thought and behavior that must be eliminated in order for a family (and the society around it) to heal and experience long-term joy, peace, and love. Most parents don't intend to pass down destructive messages to their children. In fact, most of us want more for our offspring than we had for ourselves.

Why should any of us take the time to identify our family beliefs or traditions? The reason is twofold. Doing so helps us better understand and love others, including ourselves. This is critical if you're feeling depressed. It also clearly focuses your energies on achieving your goals. Family traditions are limiting or false when they hinder your ability to love, understand, and succeed. Transcending any limiting aspects of your family's heritage increases your capacity to achieve your potential. When you are unable to love yourself, you are unable to love others. Because low self-worth sits at the core of a variety of dysfunctional behavior (for instance drug abuse, alcoholism, physical and sexual abuse, and other addictions), it is crucial to expose any limiting family teachings that may destroy your sense of worthiness.

Most limiting traditions are not spelled out consciously. Since most of what we communicate is nonverbal, families pass along what we call "non-purposeful teachings." You'd never hear someone say out loud, "In order to get love in our family you need to get straight As in school and keep a spotless room." But a parent who focuses on these things to the extreme may send the nonverbal message that a child who fails in these endeavors is not worth loving.

People who love and honor their forbearers often struggle to look objectively at their family patterns. Loving children and grandchildren often fear uncovering something negative about their relatives. They may assume that doing so will make their family appear bad, when in fact the family is good. Discovering limiting family patterns doesn't mean you've established an agenda to criticize your heritage. Rather, it gives you a chance to improve upon it.

Pay close attention to your family's attitudes, particularly to the nonverbal messages that are sent when a child behaves in a certain way. Are you passing down biases and prejudices? Or are you passing down love and acceptance? What was passed to you? How do your actions influence your children's behavior? How was your behavior influenced by your parents' actions? Spend some time writing down the answers to these questions. Discuss them with open-minded siblings, a spouse, or a friend. Simply pinpointing behaviors and attitudes that come from your family's history may be eye-opening for you and the catalyst you need to initiate change.

You may find support from Mother Nature by using white fir oil topically. White fir assists by bringing up old generational patterns that no longer serve and helping us to let them go.

MOTHER NATURE KNOWS BEST

Mother Nature rewards us for behaving in ways that support our best good. We find models discussed in each chapter of this book.

For example, when we provide the body with proper nutrition, the brain receives an increase of the neurotransmitter dopamine, a pleasure-providing neurotransmitter, suggesting to the mind and body that eating is a good idea and it will make us feel good. Of course, it is! We can't survive if we don't eat.

When we get good sleep at the appropriate times (when the sun is down), our bodies naturally regulate the neurotransmitter serotonin and the hormone melatonin—both of which are required for us to think clearly, live happy, and feel calm.

The brain is also provided with an increase in dopamine when we socially interact with others in positive ways, when we procreate, and when we come together in healthy tribal gatherings. This makes sense, too. Social interaction is necessary for our survival, and we need one another to live healthy and happy lives. Healthy family units provide a foundation for us to be happy, as it's through our families that we receive our genetic patterning, modeling for healthy attachment in relationships, and our initial belief systems. It's no wonder that we feel good when our families are functional.

Finally, the act of procreation makes human kind possible! Again, it's no wonder we are rewarded for such an act. When managed appropriately, procreation leaves our minds and bodies feeling great. Again, a nice little reward from Mother Nature to keep us doing the things that will help us not only survive, but thrive.

Mother Nature knows best. By following the messaging she's established within us, we may find that we are able to not only overcome symptoms of depression, but also resolve other health and wellness challenges.

Appendix A

Essential Oils for Treating Different Mood Conditions

The information in this section is written for educational and informational purposes. Here you will find a simple list of essential oils that can be used as a starting off point for you to begin your own research about what you can use to promote overall wellness. Such research includes working with your physician or a licensed healthcare provider to determine what is best for you. This information is not intended to replace the advice given by a healthcare professional. The essential oils listed below are not meant to replace medication or formal medical treatment. Because essential oils are *adaptogenic* (meaning, they perform many different tasks for our health), there are a variety of solutions from plants that may promote wellness. If you have any concerns about your health, particularly your mental health, we advise you to reach out to your physician. In an emergency situation, please dial 9-1-1.

Addiction

Addiction is a condition or chronic disease that affects the brain's reward and motivation circuitry. It negatively impacts brain function, overall well-being, and relationships. Addiction is debilitating, and can destroy lives. The following may help as

complementary treatment for recovery from mild addictions.
- Black pepper
- Clove
- Lavender
- Melissa
- Patchouli
- Vetiver

Anxiety

Anxiety is a feeling of nervousness or unease that can create apprehension, panic attacks, and compulsive behavior. It is sometimes a symptom of depression. The following may help as a complementary treatment for recovery from anxiety.
- Eucalyptus
- Frankincense
- Lavender
- Tangerine
- Vetiver
- Wild orange

Attention Deficit Hyperactivity Disorder (ADHD)

ADHD can be described as a neurological disorder characterized by distractibility, impulsivity, and restlessness or hyperactivity. It is often recognized in children, although it can carry into adulthood and affects the ability of these adults to find success in most aspects of life. The following may help as a complementary treatment for ADHD.
- Clary sage
- Frankincense
- Lavender
- Myrrh

- Peppermint
- Vetiver
- Ylang ylang

Depression

Depression is a state of mood that goes beyond just feeling down and blue. It's a health condition that affects thoughts, feelings of self-worth, sleep, mental focus, and more. The following may help as a complementary treatment for recovery from some forms of depression.
- Bergamot
- Frankincense
- Grapefruit
- Lime
- Melissa
- Rosemary
- Wild orange

Insomnia

Insomnia is a sleep disorder characterized by an inability to fall asleep or stay asleep. Insomnia can contribute or correlate to other mental health disorders. The following may help as a complementary treatment for recovery from insomnia.
- Clary sage
- Cedarwood
- Bergamot
- Lavender
- Roman chamomile
- Ylang ylang
- Vetiver

Menopause

Menopause is a time in a woman's life when she no longer menstruates and is no longer fertile. During this process, a woman's body undergoes many physiological changes that can affect emotional and physical well-being. The following may help as a complementary treatment for support during menopause.
- Bergamot
- Clary sage
- Cypress
- Fennel
- Geranium
- Roman chamomile

Personality Disorders

Personality disorders are deeply ingrained maladaptive disorders that typically begin in adolescence and continue into adulthood. Personality disorders typically have a long-term affect on relationships and our ability to function well in social situations.
- Bergamot
- Cypress
- Frankincense
- Grapefruit
- Lavender
- Lime
- Melissa
- White fir

Postpartum Depression

Postpartum depression is a type of clinical depression that sometimes surfaces for mothers after delivery. This form of depression is typically due to hormonal changes, fatigue, and adjustment challenges. Refer to the list of essential oils recommended for depression for support with postpartum depression.

Post-Traumatic Stress Disorder

Post traumatic stress disorder (PTSD) is a psychiatric disorder that typically results from witnessing a life-threatening trauma, undergoing an experience that threatens safety, or going through something that dramatically and destructively disrupts someone's life without warning. The following may help as complementary treatment for recovery from PTSD.
- Black pepper
- Geranium
- Helichrysum
- Lime
- Vetiver
- Wild orange

Appendix B

Essential Oils and Their Emotional Impact

The standard guidelines for emotional wellness and the relief of depression include consumption of a nutritious diet (with supplementation whenever needed), elimination of unhealthy foods and other substances from your diet and environment, adequate water intake, proper sleep habits, a resourceful outlook on life, and choosing to engage in respectful, supportive relationships. In addition, essential oils can have a positive emotional impact on you by elevating your mood, promoting relaxation, and contributing other healthful benefits.

The following list, Appendix B, is organized alphabetically by the common names of the essential oils that are mentioned. It explains emotional outcomes you can expect to experience when using each of these oils aromatically, topically, and/or internally, and some of the physical properties that may contribute to these results. *Note: The descriptions here are provided for informational purposes only, as suggestions for the kinds of results individuals may experience.*

Basil *(Ocimum basilicum)*. Basil is a member of the herb family, and as such, it has strong medicinal properties that make it an excellent choice for treating viral and bacterial infections. It is also used to treat mental exhaustion. It helps renew the mind and restore energy to the body. Basil's positive properties may help in the battle against addiction by restoring hope to the spirit.

Bergamot *(Citrus bergamia).* For those with low self-esteem, bergamot oil can restore confidence and hope. It is used to regain self-assurance, and supports letting go of negative thoughts. Bergamot encourages us with our true selves and share that with other people. It combines well with lime and sandalwood. If applied to the throat and solar plexus, it supports a sense of worthiness and belonging. A member of the citrus family, bergamot is an excellent choice for uplifting mood.

Birch *(Betula lenta).* Birch is a member of the tree family, and as such, its properties are grounding and soothing for the soul. Birch is helpful for those who feel unsupported by the people around them. When we feel alone, birch can uplift and provide comfort and strength to the spirit. It encourages us to be resilient when standing alone. It offers sustenance by helping us feel rooted enough to face the storms of life. Physically, birch provides support to the structural system of our bodies.

Black pepper *(Piper nigrum).* Black pepper is highly antiviral when taken internally, and as such, it is also powerful at eliminating the "virus" of negative thinking. Black pepper pulls up suppressed emotions and encourages recovery and new ways of thinking. It also brings up emotions so that they can be dealt with honestly. Black pepper is helpful for addiction, as it encourages letting go of old ways and increases the capacity to embrace the new. For those who bottle up emotions (such as people who express erratic behavior and addiction), black pepper may help to safely sweep out self-destructive feelings.

Cassia *(Cinnamomum cassia)*. Cassia is an oil of courage, especially useful for those who are shy and hold themselves back. By helping us to recognize our talents and potential, it enables us to replace fear with self-confidence. Cassia is medicinal in nature. It boosts the immune system and promotes circulation. It can assist in helping those who feel overrun by life to regain their inner strength. Cassia is high in cinnamaldehyde, and as such, has been shown to be useful for killing different strands of bacteria, particularly those associated with Lyme disease.

Cedarwood *(Juniperus virginiana)*. Cedarwood oil helps those who struggle with social connection. It opens the heart so we may feel the love and support of other people. It helps us to feel like we belong and eliminates our feelings of loneliness. Cedarwood belongs to the tree family, and as such, it's grounding and soothing to the central nervous system. Consequently, it can be used topically on the bottoms of the feet, along with lavender and/or Roman chamomile, to support a good night's sleep.

Cilantro *(Coriandrum sativum L.)*. Cilantro oil comes from the same plant as coriander, but is extracted in a different way—by steam extraction from the leaves. It contains antioxidants that protect our cells from oxidative stress. It also helps us cleanse ourselves of negative emotions that weigh down the body. It's a natural physical and emotional detoxifier that promotes digestion. As such, it helps us end any destructive behavior patterns we may have and lighten our emotional load, allowing us return to our true selves. Cilantro may help to treat migraine headaches and reduce heavy metal toxicity.

Cinnamon bark *(Cinnamomum zeylanicum)*. Cinnamon bark helps to regulate blood sugar. It also has antibacterial properties and is purifying to the circulatory system, as well as being good for oral health when incorporated into a mouthwash. Emotionally, it supports sexual health. It can rekindle sexual desires that have been lost because of trauma or abuse. It encourages us to be honest and vulnerable, allowing intimacy to flourish. It restores joy and well-being, and supports us in sustaining healthy boundaries in our relationships, particularly our most intimate relationships.

Clary sage *(Salvia sclarea)*. Clary sage provides clarity of mind. It helps us to open our psyches to new ideas and perspectives. It supports creativity by increasing our ability to focus and visualize. It can also help us better develop our spiritual gifts. Physically, it interacts with the body's endocrine system to bring us into hormonal balance. It stimulates our interest in intimacy. Women entering menopause may find it useful to combine clary sage with geranium (topically) to support mood and hormonal balance.

Clove *(Eugenia caryophyllata)*. Clove oil is a powerful antioxidant. It stimulates circulation and may benefit cardiovascular health. Emotionally, it supports the establishing of healthy boundaries in our relationships. It gives people with victim tendencies, who feel they can't control what's around them, a sense of personal power and control. It supports them in being able to define emotional boundaries to protect themselves.

Coriander *(Coriandrum sativum L.)*. Coriander oil comes from the same plant as cilantro, but is extracted in a different way—from the seeds. It supports balanced blood sugar levels and teaches us that we can have joy in life. Often, we grow up believing we must please others to be loved and thus, happy. When there is no joy in life at times, we may turn to sugar and sweets to make us feel better. Coriander is excellent for those who are people-pleasers and have lost sight of who they are or can't find joy in the lives they've created. It supports loyalty to ourselves by encouraging us to do the things that are in alignment with our true natures. Physically, coriander helps those with blood sugar imbalances. Therapeutic-grade coriander can be taken internally to support the body when there's been too much sugar intake. It's also useful to rub coriander directly over the pancreatic area. In addition, it may be used to treat nausea and stomach upset.

Cypress *(Cupressus sempervirens)*. Cypress oil supports the flow of energy and as such, it's tremendously useful for bringing up and releasing deeply stored pain. Individuals who feel emotionally stuck may find cypress a great resource. It encourages us to be more flexible and let go of the need to control. Physically, cypress supports the circulatory system as a vasodilator. As a member of the tree family, it provides emotional grounding and strengthens the structural systems of the body. The monoterpenes it contains stimulate localized blood flow.

Eucalyptus *(Eucalyptus radiata)*. For centuries, eucalyptus has been used to support the respiratory system. It promotes clear breathing and a healthy inflammatory response. In doing so, eucalyptus supports healing and wellness. Eucalyptus seems to tap into the emotions of those who have a pattern of illness and helps them move forward to living in wellness. It encourages us to face our issues and let go of negative emotions. Eucalyptus is grounding and soothing to the spirit and suggests a renewal of life and good health to an ailing body and spirit.

Fennel *(Foeniculum vulgare)*. Fennel aids digestive wellness and supports hormonal balance. It may ease menstrual pain when applied topically to the abdomen. It also promotes the health of the lymphatic system. Emotionally, fennel supports individuals who feel overwhelmed and reminds them of their potential. Fennel helps us reconnect with our inner selves and inspires a bigger perspective. It strengthens the soul to imagine that desires of the heart can be obtained. Just as fennel supports our physical digestion, it helps us digest the process of life.

Frankincense *(Boswellia frereana)*. Frankincense is often referred to as the "father" of essential oils. Used since antiquity, this oil helps us connect with our inner spirit. It cleanses the energy field of spiritual darkness and deception by helping us see the light within and reminding us of our talents and potential. Also, frankincense reminds us that we are loved and not forgotten. Frankincense is helpful for children and adults who struggle with issues related to a father. Soothing to the skin, it is also known to promote cellular health, a healthy inflammatory response, and boost immunity. When inhaled, it induces peace and relaxation.

Geranium *(Pelargonium graveolens)*. Geranium helps calms the nerves, lessens anxiety, and supports healthy liver functioning. It promotes hormonal balance during menopause. Geranium oil soothes a broken heart and aids in releasing emotional baggage. It helps us regain lost hope and begin to trust people and the world around us, reminding the spirit that the world is mostly good and most people have good intentions. It also brings up the pain of the past so one can work through old emotions and begin to see all that's good.

Ginger *(Zingiber officinale)*. Ginger is the ultimate encourager. Physically it promotes healthy digestion. Emotionally, it empowers individuals to fulfill the lives they were destined to create. It helps us to live in the present and seize the day. Ginger encourages the healthy processing of uncomfortable challenges and supports the resolution of gut-related anxiety.

Grapefruit *(Citrus x paradisi)*. Grapefruit is a member of the citrus family and, as such, it is a natural mood elevator. It can promote hormonal balance. It reduces mental fatigue and eliminates toxic thinking about self-worth. Historically, grapefruit has been used to reduce fat from problem areas of the body because it cleanses toxins from fatty cells. Consequently, it is a great essential oil for individuals who are unhappy with the way they look. As grapefruit oil helps us control our appetites and lose weight by stimulating healthy metabolism, it encourages us to love our bodies more. Grapefruit oil also inspires us to pay attention to what our bodies really need.

Helichrysum *(Helichrysum italicum)*. Helichrysum is known to be restorative to the skin, liver, and nervous system. It is the ultimate essential oil for healing deep emotional pain, as it helps us address emotions that are behind the pain. Helichrysum helps restore a love for life in individuals who have been weighed down by negative beliefs. It's also often useful for those struggling with addiction, self-rejection, and self-hate. Helichrysum may be useful to rub over the liver, as this is the organ that holds on to painful emotions such as anger, fear, and hate.

Juniper berry *(Juniperus communis)*. Juniper berry is often used to treat kidney and urinary tract infections. Emotionally, juniper berry helps those who are ridden by fear, anger, and a lack of security in life. Juniper berry suggests to both mind and body to work through the underlying issues creating intense fear and anger. It helps us feel protected and have the courage to face life with the knowledge that it's possible to create peace, balance, and a sense of security.

Lavender *(Lavandula augustifolia)*. Lavender is the oil of communication. It helps us open up and express our true selves honestly. It also enhances cellular communication and is a powerful anti-inflammatory. Calming and soothing to the central nervous system, lavender can dramatically reduce symptoms of anxiety. It is considered by some to be the "mother" of all essential oils, offering some of the broadest medicinal uses, from treating burns and bug bites to reducing joint pain and eliminating headaches.

Lemon *(Citrus limon)*. Lemon is a natural mood enhancer. Its clean, fresh scent brightens the environment and encourages cleanliness, as well as emotional housekeeping. Individuals who have learning disabilities or find it hard to focus may find lemon supportive. It assists us in finding clarity and choosing to live in the present, focusing on one thing at a time. It restores confidence in our ability to learn. With its high limonene content, lemon oil is a powerful antioxidant useful for detoxification and respiratory function. It is highly antibacterial and can be used as a natural hand sanitizer while uplifting mood immediately when inhaled.

Lemongrass *(Cymbopogon flexuousus)*. Lemongrass is a fantastic emotional housecleaner (assuming that the body is the house of emotions). It supports individuals who feel stagnant in life to clear the clutter and move forward. It helps energy to flow freely so we can live with confidence. Lemongrass can bridge the gap between desires of the heart and mind. Medicinally, it's helpful for bringing balance to the thyroid system. It's highly antimicrobial, anti-infectious, and helpful with increasing circulation, so it's often taken internally for overall wellness.

Lime *(Citrus aurantifolia)*. Lime, a member of the citrus family, is uplifting. High in antioxidants, it boosts immunity and supports the respiratory system. Its scent helps individuals feel joy, and reduces negative emotions such as sadness and discouragement. It instills love and happiness. It's wonderful for releasing grief and pain.

Marjoram *(Origanum majorana)*. Marjoram is a member of the herb family, and as such, it has medicinal properties; it is antibacterial and antiviral in nature. Marjoram also relieves joint and tissue pain, and promotes cardiovascular and respiratory health. It helps individuals who cannot create meaningful relationships due to emotional wounds or trauma to move forward. Marjoram may assist us in learning to trust others and ourselves more.

Melaleuca, aka tea tree *(Melaleuca alternifolia)*. An antibacterial, melaleuca promotes the integrity of the skin. It's good for cleaning. Taken internally, it boosts immunity. Emotionally, it supports us in creating strong boundaries and helps us rid ourselves of negative thoughts about others and ourselves. Melaleuca can help us stick up for what we believe in. For those who have been chronically ill, it rebuilds confidence in life and in good health.

Melissa, aka lemon balm *(Melissa officinalis)*. Melissa can cross the blood-brain barrier and is therefore powerfully supportive to the human brain. It may help us recover from traumas that have affected the brain. Highly antiviral, it is also analgesic, anti-inflammatory, antihistaminic, and antidepressant. Emotionally, melissa is sometimes referred to as the "oil of truth," as it supports us in freeing ourselves of unwanted programming that impairs healthy thinking. It supports spiritual connection. It helps us to see and understand who we really are and why we are here. It encourages us to press on through the hard times and love our lives.

Myrrh *(Commiphora myrrha)*. Myrrh boosts immunity by stimulating the production of white blood cells. Helpful for the thyroid system, myrrh is also good for digestion and helps eliminate Candida albicans. It supports healthy gums and mouth care. It can also be used at birth to help heal the cutting of an umbilical cord of a new infant. Emotionally, myrrh helps heal subconscious conflicts and encourages nurturing expression. Myrrh can help heal relationship issues, especially issues related to a hardened relationship between a mother and child. Myrrh helps the child within feel safe and loved, filling any void in childhood nurturing.

Oregano *(Origanum vulgare).* Oregano oil can relieve pain and infection. Its strong antiseptic properties work similarly to prescription antibiotics. Taken internally on a daily basis, it may help maintain healthy immunity. Oregano promotes digestion. Metaphorically, oregano oil works similarly on our emotional system, fighting for sound emotional health by helping us purify ourselves of unwanted thoughts and behaviors. It can get through to individuals who are stubborn and hold on tightly to unhealthy belief systems. Oregano aids us to let go of toxic attachments, bad relationships, and self-sabotaging habits, thus making it easier to move forward in life.

Patchouli *(Pogostemon cablin).* Patchouli is a grounding essential oil that helps stabilize the central nervous system. Its molecules can cross the blood-brain barrier. Some people find it gives them relief from headache symptoms. It helps connect the heart and body so that they can work better together. It also supports us in letting go of negative thoughts about life and reminds us to find beauty in the world around us. Patchouli can aid in addiction recovery, as it helps us to shift our attitudes and establish a healthy connection to life.

Peppermint *(Mentha piperita).* Peppermint stimulates the brain and increases circulation. It is good for headaches, memory, and focusing. To rapidly improve mood and enhance brain function, combine with wild orange and inhale. As you do so, you'll find you've increased neuronal activity in your brain (you'll also open up your sinus membranes), and suddenly you'll feel a wave of happy emotions encompassing you. Emotionally, peppermint helps individuals struggling with depression to see the joy in life. Peppermint reduces pressure and can put a cap on an overflow of unhealthy emotions.

Roman Chamomile *(Anthemus nobilis).* Roman chamomile is calming to mind and body, aids digestion (and relieves colic in infants), and promotes a healthy inflammatory response. Emotionally, it can help us feel a renewed sense of purpose or heal a broken heart. Roman chamomile gives confidence and motivation to succeed or go on. It helps us process our emotions.

Rose *(Rosa damascena).* Rose promotes skin elasticity and wound healing. It has many spiritual purposes as well. It encourages spiritual healing by helping us sense divine love. When we can connect to divine love, our emotional wounds tend to resolve. Rose aids prayer and meditation. It helps us feel more compassion and charity. Rose brings spiritual clarity and can be useful during birth and death transitions, bringing great peace and comfort.

Rosemary *(Rosmarinus officinalis).* Rosemary may improve adrenal fatigue and mental exhaustion. It promotes respiratory function, digestion, memory, and learning. Emotionally, rosemary encourages us to gain greater knowledge by searching for deeper answers. It helps us to expand our minds beyond first assumptions. Rosemary also helps us feel comfortable and confident in times of change. It lightens our sense of being emotionally burdened.

Sandalwood *(Santalum album).* Research on sandalwood suggests that it has powerful properties that aid in restoring cellular function. Sandalwood helps to calm the heart and prepares us to talk to God. It is an aid to meditation. Sandalwood assists us in opening the soul to honest and healthy connection. In doing so, it offers clarity and spiritual strengthening. It also allows us to see life from a bigger perspective. It can help us better align our lives with divine purpose.

Tangerine *(Citrus reticulata)*. Tangerine is a member of the citrus family, and as such, it is a natural mood enhancer. It is antiseptic and stimulates red blood-cell production, improving the oxygen-carrying capacity of the blood. It soothes inflammation and promotes circulation and excretion of toxic substances. Emotionally, tangerine frees us to let go of even the most debilitating of pressures for a period, and to be happy. It helps us to restore creativity.

Tea tree *(see Melaleuca)*.

Thyme *(Thymus vulgaris CT Thymol)*. A member of the herb family, thyme is an antimicrobial. It is also a powerful antioxidant and analgesic. Emotionally, thyme helps release buried feelings, including resentment that's been stored for a long time. Bringing unhealthy emotions to the surface helps us process, and ultimately get rid of them. By ridding our minds and bodies of strongly rooted negative emotions, we can create better health, confidence, and emotional fortitude.

Vetiver *(Vetiveria zizanioides)*. Vetiver is tremendously soothing for the multitasking mind that tends to gravitate toward distraction and other symptoms of ADHD. It helps balance the mind and creates mental clarity for those torn between people or priorities, and those who have trouble making simple decisions. Vetiver smells like earth, and grounds us by helping us connect to ourselves. It gives us confidence to know what to do, when, and why. It improves sleep, enhances focus and attention, and helps us release thoughts of painful trauma.

White fir *(Abies alba)*. White fir is a natural painkiller. It belongs to the tree family, and so is grounding. It also enhances respiration and relaxes the body while stimulating the mind. This makes white fir especially suitable for healing unhealthy generational patterns and emotional wounds. Of the emotions passed down by family members, some are good and some, such as addiction, pride, and codependency, are destructive. White fir brings beliefs to the surface of our conscious minds so that we can work through them and break destructive patterns.

Wild orange *(Citrus sinensis).* High in monoterpenes, wild orange is an immune booster and antioxidant. It promotes circulation and liver detoxification. As a member of the citrus family, it is mood uplifting and encourages happiness. Wild orange helps us rid our minds of fear and anxiety. It reminds the spirit of the innate presence of universal bliss.

Wintergreen *(Gaultheria procumbens).* Wintergreen is a painkiller. Because it contains methyl salicylate, it soothes joint pain and muscle soreness. It promotes respiration and mental clarity. For those who inhale it, it may also help relieve emotional pain. Wintergreen helps us let go of negative energy, and teaches us that we do not need to carry our burdens alone and do not always need to be right. With its help, we may be able to stop carrying the burdens of wrongdoing by others and release the pain associated with our past trials.

Ylang ylang *(Cananga odorata).* Ylang ylang oil is effective in treating infections of the gastrointestinal tract. It can bring relief from tachycardia (rapid heart beat), heart palpitations, and hypertension. It brings euphoria and soothes inflammation. Emotionally, ylang ylang helps us open our hearts and bring security to the inner child. It suggests that it is safe to be open to feeling love and joy. Consequently, ylang ylang can assist people who have gone through intense emotional trauma, helping them to let go of the pain and move forward in life.

Acknowledgements

I would like to express my deepest appreciation to my dear friend and cowriter, Stephanie Gunning. Without a doubt, Stephanie is one of the most talented editors and authors of our time. Her breadth of knowledge about health and wellness, and her sharp ability to refine a topic and present it in book form is simply unprecedented. I am grateful that she accepted the last-minute challenge to help me create and refine this message.

I am always most grateful to my dear husband, Shane Hintze, my best friend and the person I dedicated this book to. I've learned some of my most valuable lessons with Shane by my side. Year after year, he provides emotional, spiritual, and physical support, allowing me to grow and thrive. I expect to spend eternity with this man, and that makes me happy!

Many thanks must be given to my beautiful children, Ashley, Nick, Katie, and Michael. Without them, our lives would be empty and the fullness of our potential would not be met. Each is inspiring and they have taught us much about life and happiness. We have found that our greatest joy comes through our posterity.

Year in and year out, I am blessed with an extended family to hold me up. I am forever grateful to my mother, Nancy Linder, who taught me about mothering, nurturing, thriving, surviving, and most importantly, loving. I would seat her among the best mothers ever to walk the Earth. Her friendship and support means everything. She brought into this world my "pretty sisters," who are my dearest friends and greatest supporters, Martha Montagnoli and Callie Steuer. And she gifted me with the finest of brothers, Richard and Robert Linder. We called ourselves the "club" growing up, and my membership in the "club" means everything.

Thanks must be given to Quinn Curtis, an extraordinarily talented graphic designer and branding specialist. Her work, along with the graphic talent of Gus Yoo, made this book lovely. Thanks also to eagle-eyed proofreader Claire Putsche at Lincoln Square Books. I am grateful to Connie Higley at AromaTools for her continued support retailing books that help so many to grow. And a big thank you to Barry Merrill at Alexander's for orchestrating the printing of so many of my projects.

I express thanks to the executives at dōTERRA Corporation as they supported my research into their Lifelong Vitality product. I am grateful for all I've learned from Dr. David Hill, D.C., Chief Medical Advisor and Chairman of the Scientific Advisory Board at dōTERRA. I am grateful for the knowledge I've gained from my association with Dr. Susan Lawton, my coauthor of *Living Healthy and Happily Ever After*. I'm grateful for my friendship with Laura Jacobs. She has shared the message of healing families with me and along side me for decades. She has taught me much! And I am grateful for my longtime friend, Connie Boucher, for insisting that I purchase a box of essential oils from her in 2008. She changed my life on that hot summer day, and I am thankful.

To all my friends and associates at dōTERRA, may this book support your efforts to share a message of hope and wellness to those who are depressed or struggling with mental health issues. I am grateful for your efforts to make the world a better place.

Notes

Introduction: Overcoming Depression Naturally

1. "Depression: Fact Sheet No. 329," World Health Organization (October 2012). Available at: http://www.who.int/mediacentre/factsheets/fs369/en

2. U.S. National Institutes of Health statistic cited in R. Kessler et al. "Prevalence, Severity, and Comorbidity of Twelve-month DSM-IV Disorders in the National Comorbidity Survey Replication (NCS-R)," *Archives of General Psychiatry*, vol. 62, no. 6 (June 2005): pp. 617–27.

3. U.K. Office of National Statistics cited in A. Self et al, 2012), "Measuring National Well-being: Life in the UK," Office for National Statistics, (November 2012).

4. "Depression: Fact Sheet No. 329."

5. H. J. Kang et al. "Decreased Expression of Synapse-related Genes and Loss of Synapses in Major Depressive Disorder," *Nature Medicine*, vol. 18 (2012): pp. 1413–7.

6. Kathlyn Stone. "The Changing Face of the Anti-Depressant Drug Market," About Money (accessed August 2014). Available at: http://pharma.about.com/od/Sales_and_Marketing/a/The-Changing-Face-Of-The-Anti-Depressant-Drug-Market.htm

7. A.A. Nierenberg et al. "The Current Crisis of Confidence in Antidepressants," *Journal of Clinical Psychiatry*, vol. 72 (2011): pp. 27–33.

8. Andrew Stanway. *Overcoming Depression* (London: Hamlyn Publishing Group, 1981).

9. B.T. Walsh et al. (2002). "Placebo Response in Studies of Major Depression: Variable, Substantial, and Growing," *Journal of the American Medical Association*, vol. 287, no. 14 (April 2002): pp. 1840–7.

10. M.E. Thase. "Effectiveness of Antidepressants: Comparative Remission Rates," *Journal of Clinical Psychiatry*, vol. 64 (2003): pp. 3–7.

11. "Selective Serotonin Reuptake Inhibitors (SSRIs), Mayo Clinic (posted July 9, 2013). Available at: http://www.mayoclinic.org/diseases-conditions/depression/in-depth/ssris/art-20044825

12. Simon N. Young. "How to Increase Serotonin in the Human Brain Without Drugs," *Journal of Psychiatry Neuroscience*, vol. 32, no. 6 (2007): pp. 394–99.

13. P. Holford. "Depression: The Nutrition Connection," *Primary Care Mental Health*, vol. 1 (2003): pp. 9–16.

Mother Nature's Answer 1: Happy Nutrition

1. T. Baldwin and M. Lapointe. "The Chemistry of Amino Acids," Biology Project [online] (2003). Available at: http://www.biology.arizona.edu/biochemistry/problem_sets/aa/aa.html

2. Ibid.

3. M. Maes et al. "Hypozincemia in Depression," *Journal of Affective Disorders*, vol. 31, no. 2 (1994): p. 13.

4. Emily Deans. "Zinc! An Antidepressant?" Evolutionary Psychiatry [blog] (posted September 15, 2013). Available at: http://www.psychologytoday.com/blog/evolutionary-psychiatry/201309/zinc-antidepressant

5. Lawrence, Wilson, "Copper Toxicity," Healing Edge Sciences (accessed August 2014). Available at: http://www.healingedge.net/store/article_copper_toxicity.html

6. "Iron and Iron Deficiency," Centers for Disease Control and Prevention (accessed August 2014). Available at: http://www.cdc.gov/nutrition/everyone/basics/vitamins/iron.html

7. "Magnesium: Fact Sheet for Health Professionals," National Institutes of Health, Office of Dietary Supplements (accessed August 2014). Available at: http://ods.od.nih.gov/factsheets/Magnesium-HealthProfessional

8. Daniel K. Hall-Flavin. "What's the Relationship Between Vitamin B-12 and Depression?" Mayo Clinic (accessed August 2014). Available at: http://www.mayoclinic.org/diseases-conditions/depression/expert-answers/vitamin-b12-and-depression/faq-20058077

9. "Vitamin B6: Fact Sheet for Consumers," National Institutes of Health, Office of Dietary Supplements (accessed August 2014). Available at: http://ods.od.nih.gov/factsheets/VitaminB6-Consumer

10. "Folate," The World's Healthiest Foods (accessed August 2014). Available at: http://www.whfoods.com/genpage.php?tname=nutrient&dbid=63

11. "Omega 3 Fatty Acids," Cleveland Clinic (posted October 2013). Available at: http://my.clevelandclinic.org/heart/prevention/nutrition/food-choices/omega-3-fatty-acids.aspx

12. Tyler Graham and Drew Ramsey. T*he Happiness Diet: A Nutritional Prescription for a Sharp brain, Balanced Mood, and Lean, Energized Body* (New York: Rodale, 2001): p. 75.

13. David Pacchioli. "The Joy of Garlic" Penn State News (posted May 1, 1999). Available at: http://news.psu.edu/story/141553/1999/05/01/research/joy-garlic

14. "Kyolic® Aged Garlic Extract™," AIM Canada (posted 2009). Available at: http://www.theaimcompanies.com/datasheets/3/85E.pdf

15. J. Sanmukhani et al. "Efficacy and Safety of Curcumin in Major Depressive Disorder," *Phytotherapy Research*, vol. 28, no. 4 (April 2014: pp. 579–85.

16. A. Sánchez-Villegas et al. "Fast-Food and Commercial Baked Goods Consumption and the Risk of Depression," *Public Health Nutrition*, vol. 15, no. 3 (March 2012): pp 424–32.

17. Ibid.

18. Carson Boddicker. "Brain Derived Neurotrophic Factor and Exercise," LiveStrong (posted August 16, 2013). Available at: http://www.livestrong.com/article/214646-brain-derived-neurotrophic-factor-exercise

19. William Dufty. "Refined Sugar: The Sweetest Poison of All" Global Healing Center (accessed August 2014). Available at: http://www.globalhealingcenter.com/sugar-problem/refined-sugar-the-sweetest-poison-of-all

20. Kris Gunnars. "Top 13 Evidence-based Health Benefits of Coffee," Authority Nutrition (accessed August 2014). Available at: http://authoritynutrition.com/top-13-evidence-based-health-benefits-of-coffee

21. Patrick Cameron. "Depression Caused by Liver Disease," Live Strong (posted August 16, 2013). Available at: http://www.livestrong.com/article/17243-depression-caused-liver-disease

22. Elizabeth Lipski, *Digestive Wellness: How to Strengthen the Immune System and Prevent Diseases Through Healthy Digestion* (New York: McGraw-Hill, 2005): p. 217.

23. "SAM-e (S-adenosylmethionine, SAMe)," WebMD (accessed August 2014). Available at: http://www.webmd.com/vitamins-and-supplements/lifestyle-guide-11/supplement-guide-sam-e

24. "Milk Thistle Supplement for Depression Anxiety" Depression Anxiety Diet [blog] (posted February 22, 2013). Available at: http://www.depressionanxietydiet.com/milk-thistle-supplementfor-depression-anxiety

25. V. Bansal et al. "Stimulating the Central Nervous System to Prevent Intestinal Dysfunction after Traumatic Brain Injury," *Journal of Trauma*, vol. 68, no 5 (2010): pp. 1059–64.

26. Adam Hadhazy. "Think Twice: How the Gut's 'Second Brain' Influences Mood and Well-Being" Scientific American (February 12, 2010). Available at: http://www.scientificamerican.com/article/gut-second-brain

27. Ibid.

28. Gisela Telis. "Can What You Eat Affect Your Mental Health?" *Washington Post* (March 24, 2014). Available at: http://www.washingtonpost.com/national/health-science/can-what-you-eat-affect-your-mental-health-new-research-links-diet-and-the-mind/2014/03/24/c6b40876-abc0-11e3-af5f-4c56b834c4bf_story.html

29. K. Tillisch et al. "Consumption of Fermented Milk Product with Probiotic Modulates Brain Activity," *Gastroenterology*, vol. 1444, no 7 (June 2013): pp. 1394–401.

30. J. Licinio and M. L. Wong. "The Role of Inflammatory Mediators in the Biology of Major Depression," *Molecular Psychiatry*, vol. 4 (1999): pp. 317–27.

31. Lipski: p. 68.

32. Jill Grunewald. "13 Ways to Treat Hypothyroidism Naturally," MindBodyGreeen.com (posted September 15, 2011). Available at: http://www.mindbodygreen.com/0-3139/13-Ways-to-Treat-Hypothyroidism-Naturally.html

Mother Nature's Answer 2: Happy Lifestyle

1. Roni Caryn Rabin. "New Worries About Sleeping Pills," *New York Times* (March 12, 2012). Available at: http://well.blogs.nytimes.com/2012/03/12/new-worries-about-sleeping-pills

2. David DiSalvo. "To Get More Sleep, Get More Sunlight" Frobes.com (posted June 18, 2013). Available at: http://www.forbes.com/sites/daviddisalvo/2013/06/18/to-get-more-sleep-get-more-sunlight

3. Virgil D. Wooten. "How to Fall Asleep: Sunlight and Sleep," How Stuff Works (accessed August 2014). Available at: http://health.howstuffworks.com/mental-health/sleep/basics/how-to-fall-asleep2.htm

4. *Reset Your Inner Clock: The Drug-free Way to Your Best-ever Sleep, Mood, and Energy*, by Michael Terman and Ian McMahan (New York: Avery, 2013).

5. Maysan Marouf. "Why Sunlight Is the Best Anti-depressant," *Mystera* (accessed August 2014). Available at: http://mystera-magazine.com/article/why-sunshine-best-anti-depressant

6. Ibid.

7. "Chronic Stress Puts Your Health at Risk," Mayo Clinic (posted July 11, 2013). Available at: http://www.mayoclinic.org/healthy-living/stress-management/in-depth/stress/art-20046037

8. "Stress Responses," Valley City State University (accessed August 2014). Available at: http://www.vcsu.edu/cmsfiles/75/stress_r_bteu67.pdf

9. "Parasympathetic Nervous System," Wikipedia (accessed August 2014). Available at: http://en.wikipedia.org/wiki/Parasympathetic_nervous_system

10. Herbert Benson with Miriam Z. Klipper. *The Relaxation Response.* (New York: HarperTorch, 2000): pp. 162-3.

11. "Mindfulness Meditation Is Associated With Structural Changes in the Brain," National Center for Complementary and Alternative Medicine (NCCAM), National Institutes of Health (January 30, 2011). Available at: http://nccam.nih.gov/research/results/spotlight/012311.htm

12. Kellie Marksberry. "Take a Deep Breath," American Institute of Stress (posted August 10, 2012). Available at: http://www.stress.org/take-a-deep-breath

13. Candace B. Pert. "Letter to the Editor," Time (October 20, 1997): p. 8.

14. K. Pilkington et al. "Yoga for Depression: The Research Evidence," *Journal of Affective Disorders,* vol. 89, no. 1-3 (December 2005): pp. 13-24.

15. Chris Illiades and Pat F. Bass. "Yoga as Depression treatment," Everyday Health (posted June 23, 2011). Available at: Everydayhealth.com/depression/yoga-as-depression-treatment.aspx

16. Meera Balasubramaniam et al. "Yoga on Our Minds," Frontiers in Psychiatry (January 25, 2013). Available at: http://www.frontiersin.org/Affective_Disorders_and_Psychosomatic_Research/10.3389/fpsyt.2012.00117/abstract

17. Andrea L. Dunn et al. "Exercise Treatment for Depression," *American Journal of Preventive Medicine*, vol. 28, no. 1 (January 2005): pp. 1-8.

18. Y. Li et al. "Long-term Tai Chi Training Is Related to Depressive Symptoms Among Tai Chi Practitioners," *Journal of Affective Disorders* (July 31, 2014): pp. 36-9.

19. Sarah Novotny and Len Kravitz, Ph.D. "The Science of Breathing," University of New Mexico (accessed August 2014). Available at: http://www.unm.edu/~lkravitz/Article%20folder/Breathing.html

20. Sameer A. Zope and Rakesh A Zope. "Sudarshan Kriya Yoga: Breathing for Health," International Journal of Yoga, vol. 6, no. 1 (January-June 2013): pp. 4-10. Available at: http://www.ncbi.nlm.nih.gov/pmc/articles/PMC3573542

21. K. Aleisha Fetters. "How to Achieve a Runner's High: Science Reveals How You Can Produce More Feel-Good Chemicals While Running," *Runners World* (April 25, 2014). Available at: http://www.runnersworld.com/running-tips/how-to-achieve-a-runners-high.

22. Ibid.

23. Dharmendra Solanki and Andrew M. Lane, "Relationships Between Exercise as a Mood Regulation Strategy and Trait Emotional Intelligence," *Asian Journal of Sports Medicine*, vol. 1, no. 4 (December 2010): pp. 195-200.

24. B.G. Berger and R.W. Motl. "Exercise and Mood: A Selective Review and Synthesis of Research Employing the Profile of Mood States," *Journal of Applied Sport Psychology*, vol. 12 (2000): pp. 69–92.

25. James Gordon, as cited in Joseph Mercola. "Please Don't Visit This Type of Doctor Unless You Absolutely Have to," Mercola.com (March 7, 2011). Available at: http://articles.mercola.com/sites/articles/archive/2011/03/07/reversing-depression-without-antidepressants.aspx

26. Michael Grant White. "Depression and Breathing," Optimal Breathing Mastery (accessed August 2014). Available at: http://www.breathing.com/articles/depression.htm

Mother Nature's Answer 3: Happy Relationships

1. Carl G. Jung, from his presidential address, *"Psychological Aspects of the Mother Archetype,"* which opened the Tenth International Medical Congress for Psychotherapy held July 30–August 6, 1938, at Oxford University.

2. Daniel Goleman. *Emotional Intelligence: Why It Can Matter More Than IQ* (New York: Bantam, 1995).

3. Peter Salovey and John Mayer. An article, "Emotional Intelligence" (1990), posted on a University of New Hampshire Emotional Intelligence website (accessed Augsut 2014). Available at: http://www.unh.edu/emotional_intelligence/EI%20Assets/Reprints...EI%20Proper/EI1990%20Emotional%20Intelligence.pdf

4. James W. Pennebaker. "Writing about Emotional Experiences as a Therapeutic Process, Psychological Science, vol. 8, no. 3 (May 1997): pp. 162–6.

5. Ibid.

6. Deepak Chopra, "Healing from Depression," Chopra Centered Lifestyle [blog] (accessed August 2014.) Available at: http://www.chopra.com/ccl/healing-from-depression
7. Kyla Stinnett, editor. "Rewire Your Brain for Happiness," *Chopra Center Newsletter* [online] (April 12, 2012). Available at: http://www.chopra.com/files/newsletter/Apr12/Apr12-Meditation.html
8. Candace Pert. *Molecules of Emotion: The Science Behind Mind-Body Medicine* (New York: Scribner, 1997).
9. Ibid.
10. Ibid.
11. Shahrookh Khani1 et al. "A Comparison of Adaptive and Maladaptive Perfectionists and Non-perfectionists," European Journal of Experimental Biology, vol. 3, no. 2 (2013): pp. 608–12.
12. Nelson Mandela, *Conversations with Myself* (New York: Farrar, Straus and Giroux, 2010): p. 211.
13. Deepak Chopra. *Seven Spiritual Laws of Success: A Practical Guide to the Fulfillment of Your Dreams* (San Rafael, CA.: Amber-Allyn Publishing, 1994).
14. Ibid.
15. Brent Q. Hafen et al. *The Health Effects of Attitudes, Emotions, Relationships* (Provo, UT.: EMS Asscoiates, 1992).
16. Ibid.
17. Ashley Montagu. *Touching: The Human Significance of the Skin* (New York: HarperCollins Publishers, 1971).
18. Xian Zhang et al. "Can Depression Be Diagnosed by

Response to Mother's Face? A Personalized Attachment-based Paradigm for Diagnostic fMRI," *PLoS ONE* (December 13, 2011). Available at: http://www.plosone.org/article/info%3Adoi%2F10.1371%2Fjournal.pone.0027253

19. Ibid.

20. M. Kosfeld et al. "Oxytocin Increases Trust in Humans," Nature, vol. 435, no. 7042 (June 2005): pp. 673–6. Also: Paul J. Zak et al. "Oxytocin Increases Generosity in Humans," PLoS ONE, vol. 2, no. 11 (November 7, 2007): p. e1128; and Angela A. Stanton. "Neural Substrates of Decision-making in Economic Games," *Scientific Journals International*, vol. 1, no. 1 (2007): pp. 1–64.

21. P. Kirsch et al. "Oxytocin Modulates Neural Circuitry for Social Cognition and Fear in Humans," *Journal of Neuroscience*, vol. 25, no. 49 (December 2005): pp. 11489–93.

22. "Stress Responses," Valley City State University (accessed August 2014). Available at: http://www.vcsu.edu/cmsfiles/75/stress_r_bteu67.pdf

23. Quotables.com.

24. Gregg Braden, *The Divine Matrix: Bridging Time, Space, Miracles, and Belief* (Carlsbad, CA.: Hay House, 2007): pp. 67–8.

Recommended Resources

Rebecca Hintze

www.EssentiallyHappy.com

SUPPLIERS of ESSENTIAL OILS TOOLS

AromaTools
AromaTools.com

My Oil Business
MyOilBusiness.com

READING on NUTRITION

Digestive Wellness: How to Strengthen the Immune System and Prevent Diseases Through Healthy Digestion, by Elizabeth Lipski (McGraw-Hill, 2005).

The Happiness Diet: A Nutritional Prescription for a Sharp Brain, Balanced Mood, and Lean, Energized Body, by Tyler Graham and Drew Ramsey (Rodale, 2001).

Salt, Sugar, Fat: How the Food Giants Hooked Us, by Michael Moss (Random House, 2013).

Stop Aging Now! The Ultimate Plan for Staying Young and Reversing the Aging Process, by Jean Carper (HarperCollins, 1995).

Sugar Blues, by William Dufty (Warner Books, 1993).

READING on ESSENTIAL OILS

Emotions and Essential Oils: A Modern Resource for Healing, second edition, by Daniel McDonald (Enlighten, 2013).

Living Healthy and Happily Ever After, by Rebecca Linder Hintze and Dr. Susan Lawton (Living HEA, 2012)

Modern Essentials: A Contemporary Guide to the Therapeutic Use of Essential Oils, fifth edition (AromaTools, 2013).

READING on LIFESTYLE

Whiff! The Revolution of Scent Communication in the Information Age, by C. Russell Brumfield with James Goldney and Stephanie Gunning (Quimby Press, 2008).

The Relaxation Response, by Herbert Benson (William Morrow, 1975).

Reset Your Inner Clock: The Drug-free Way to Your Best-ever Sleep, Mood, and Energy, by Michael Terman and Ian McMahan (Avery, 2013).

READING on EMOTIONS & BELIEFS

The Biology of Belief: Unleashing the Power of Consciousness, Matter, and Miracles, by Bruce H. Lipton (Hay House, 2008).

The Divine Matrix: Bridging Time, Space, Miracles, and Belief, by Gregg Braden (Hay House, 2007).

Emotional Intelligence: Why It Can Matter More Than IQ, by Daniel Goleman (Bantam, 1995).

Molecules of Emotion: The Science Behind Mind-Body Medicine, by Candace B. Pert (Scribner, 1997).

Second Firsts: Live, Laugh, and Love Again, by Christina Rasmussen (Hay House, 2013).

READING on RELATIONSHIPS

Healing Your Family History: 5 Steps to Break Free of Destructive Patterns, by Rebecca Linder Hintze (Hay House, 2006).

Social Intelligence: The New Science of Human Relationships, by Daniel Goleman (Bantam, 2006).

SUPPORT ORGANIZATIONS

Anxiety and Depression Association of America
ADAA.org

Aromatic Science
AromaticScience.com

Depression and Bipolar Support Alliance
DBSAlliance.org

Mental Health America
MentalHealthAmerica.org

National Alliance on Mental Illness
NAMI.org

National Institute of Mental Health/National Institutes of Health
NIMH.nih.gov

Postpartum Support International
PostPartum.net

About the Author

Rebecca Linder Hintze, M.Sc., is a family issues expert and bestselling author of *Healing Your Family History* (Hay House, 2006), which has been translated in eight languages, and *Living Healthy and Happily Ever After* with Dr. Susan Lawton (Living HEA, 2012). She holds a bachelor's degree from Brigham Young University and a master's degree from University of East London, School of Psychology.

Rebecca specializes in helping individuals break free of destructive family patterns. To this purpose, she has worked for nearly two decades, completing thousands of private sessions. As a speaker, Rebecca lectures on healing family patterns, overcoming destructive behavior, resolving family conflict, and treating health care issues naturally using essential oils and supplementation. A former broadcast journalist, Rebecca makes frequent appearances on television and radio.

Rebecca has been married for more than twenty-five years to Shane Hintze, and together they have four grown children and one grandson. She resides in Northern Virginia.

About the Cowriter

Stephanie Gunning is an internationally acclaimed mind-body-spirit writer, editor, and strategist whose work has contributed to the success in publishing of many of the most popular and well-recognized spiritual and personal growth thought leaders of our era, among them several *New York Times* bestselling authors. As a consultant, editor, and writer, her clients have included major publishing firms, top caliber literary agencies, and innovative self-publishers. She has mastered the art of transforming powerful ideas into marketable books.

In addition to coauthoring and ghostwriting dozens of books, Stephanie is cofounder of Lincoln Square Books, a New York-based project management and book packaging firm serving the editorial, production, and marketing needs of authors who independently publish.

Stephanie resides in New York City.

Nutrition and Depression: The Effects of dōTERRA's Lifelong Vitality Pack on Depression and Anxiety

Rebecca Linder Hintze, M.Sc.

Abstract

Objectives: This research constitutes a preliminary investigation into the effects on people's mood of a potent nutritional supplement pack called Lifelong Vitality (LLV) marketed for daily use by dōTERRA Corporation. This nutritional supplement pack contains vitamins and minerals, essential fatty acids, polyphenols, and other nutritional energy co-factors that are shown to support optimal health.

Design: This study design comprises a single group of participants self-declared as having been diagnosed with a mood disorder (i.e., depression or anxiety). A repeated measures design was used to evaluate mood as the dependent variable using the following measures: 1) Hospital Anxiety and Depression Scale (HADS), 2) General Health Questionnaire (GHQ-12), 3) Center for Epidemiological Studies Depression Scale (CES-D), and 4) Perceived Stress Scale (PSS). Time constituted the independent variable and had four levels: Each of the four measures were taken prior to commencing usage of LLV and at weekly intervals thereafter until conclusion of the study 60 days later.

Methods: Twenty-one participants (ages 18 or older, of any nationality, living in the UK) diagnosed with depression or anxiety and not taking medication were given Lifelong Vitality Pack for 60 days (participants who had recently stopped taking medication for depression were eligible to participate in this study). All participants had no prior usage of LLV. At the beginning and end of the study, and on a weekly basis, participants anonymously answered questionnaires from selected measures to determine if the supplement pack affected their mood. Data was collected online through smartsurvey.co.uk, downloaded to Excel, and uploaded for statistical analysis using IBM SPSS.

Results: A repeated measures ANOVA with 'time' as the repeated measure, followed by statistically controlled pair-wise comparisons, found significant or near significant improvements in mood across all four measures: HADS ($P<0.04$), GHQ-12 ($P<0.0001$), CES-D ($P<0.041$) and a tendency for PSS ($P<0.07$).

Conclusions: dōTERRA's Lifelong Vitality Pack may have improved mood over time and the results may be from dōTERRA's LLV product; however, some additional factors would have to be incorporated into the design in order to further test the role of dōTERRA's LLV more completely. These are preliminary findings and further research is recommended.

Introduction

Depression is one of the largest problems our world faces today. It is rated by the World Health Organization as the leading cause of disease burden among high-income countries. In the US, the National Institute of Health reports that 25 percent of the population suffers from depression (Kessler, 2005). This trend in mental health is not estimated to change in the near future. According to the *Institute of Functional Medicine,* depression is projected to be the second leading cause of disability worldwide by 2020.

Depression is typically diagnosed on the basis of symptoms and can be determined (in part) from a self-report questionnaire test (Radloff,1977). These self-report tests generally contain questions about mood, emotions, suicidal thoughts, insomnia, agitation, anxiety, stress, and so on. Depending on symptoms and test scores, these questionnaires may help practitioners diagnose the severity of depression.

Depression is generally described as a chemical imbalance, but such a diagnosis encompasses a complex umbrella of possible causes to explain such an imbalance. There are millions, even billions, of chemical reactions that make up the dynamic system responsible for mood, perceptions, and how life is experienced.

Antidepressant medications are the most common form of treatment for depression today. The annual costs of antidepressants in 1985 were $240 million in the United States. More recently, that number has jumped to $12 billion (Zorc, 2001). Even though antidepressants are widely prescribed by doctors, cases of depression continue to increase, suggesting that antidepressant medications are not working as well as expected. Some scholars have alluded to this trend as "a crisis of confidence in antidepressants" (Nierenberg, 2011). In his book Overcoming Depression, Dr. Andrew Stanway, a British physician, says "If anti-depressant drugs were really as effective as they are made out to be, surely hospital admission rates for depression would have fallen over the twenty years they've been available. Alas, this has not happened. . . . Many trials have found that tricyclics are only marginally more effective than placebos, and some have even found that they are not as effective as dummy tablets" (1981). Some twenty years after Dr. Stanway's conclusions were published, researchers looked through the results of 75 studies in which participants were randomly selected to receive either a placebo or the antidepressant under review. The results were revealing: "The response to placebo in published trials of antidepressant medication for MDD is highly variable and often substantial and has increased significantly in recent years, as has the response to medication. These observations support the view that the inclusion of a placebo group has major scientific importance in trials of new antidepressant medications and indicate that efforts should continue to minimize the risks of such studies so that they may be conducted in an ethically acceptable manner" (Walsh, 2002). The fact that studies continue to demonstrate variable successes with a placebo indicates a need for continuing research into how antidepressants are tested and against what standards.

Existing drugs are effective in only half of patients with depression (Thase, 2003). Furthermore, these drugs can take three to four weeks before their beneficial effects are manifest. And, as with all drugs, there are a number of side effect issues. Dr. Michael E. Thase, in his review of remission rates in clinical studies for antidepressants, describes why a 50 percent remission rate just isn't good enough. "A 50% reduction in depressive symptoms may be a reliable indicator of treatment response in clinical trials, but it is an inadequate goal for the initial phase of therapy. Remission, i.e., the virtual elimination of depressive symptoms and restoration of psychosocial capabilities, is fast becoming the criterion by which antidepressants are measured" (2003). If an antidepressant cannot achieve absolute elimination of symptoms, other avenues must be explored, including nutritional supplements, the placebo effect, exercise, and therapy.

Over the past two decades, research has begun to point to nutritional imbalances as contributors to depression, particularly the lack of essential fatty acids, imbalanced homocysteine levels, imbalanced serotonin levels caused by lack of amino acids, blood sugar imbalance, imbalanced levels of the nutrients chromium and Vitamin D, and food intolerances (Holford, 2003). A vast number of studies have looked at depression and how it affects mood, behaviour, and, of course, physical health. Not all studies indicate direct correlations between mood and nutrition; but nearly all of them present evidence that further study in this area could provide breakthrough results in treating depression, as well as a slew of other mental disabilities.

This research explores the effects of nutrition on depression and anxiety and studies whether or not nutritional supplementation via dōTERRA's Lifelong Vitality (LLV) pack could be an adequate treatment for depression. Lifelong Vitality Pack is a comprehensive, multi-component dietary supplement that has been formulated to contain vitamins and minerals, essential fatty acids, poly-phenols, and other nutritional energy co-factors that are shown to support optimal health (Parker, 2013). Moreover, LLV has been reported by its users to increase mood and improve mental focus (Parker, 2013).

This study involves a preliminary evaluation to determine the before and after effects of dōTERRA's Lifelong Vitality daily nutritional supplement pack (LLV) on four clinical measures of depression (i.e., HADS, GHQ-12, CES-D, PSS) following 60 days of supplementation in individuals diagnosed with depression and currently without anti-depressant medication.

Materials and Methods

Participants: Notice for participants for this study was broadcast through word of mouth, an announcement to a local London Christian church group, and UK distributors of dōTERRA products. Twenty-one participants (15 women and 6 men ages

18 or older, of any nationality, living in the UK) diagnosed with depression and not taking medication were given Lifelong Vitality Pack for 60 days (participants who recently stopped medication for depression were eligible to participate in this study). All participants had no prior usage of LLV.

Lifelong Vitality Pack: Lifelong Vitality Pack (LLV) includes three bottled supplements: Alpha CRS+®, xEO Mega, and Microplex VMz®. Lifelong Vitality Pack was released in 2008 and has undergone minor updates in content since that time. These products are packaged in separate bottles but are contained in one box. There are no known side effects from taking dōTERRA's Lifelong Vitality Pack; the product is wheat free and dairy free. dōTERRA LLV is sold in the UK, and the company has a European office in London. Participants were shipped a one-time supply of LLV to cover the extent of the study (i.e., 2 months or 60 days) and were asked to follow the manufacturer's instructions for daily dosage. The ingredients are generally described by dōTERRA as follows:

Alpha CRS+® CELLULAR VITALITY COMPLEX
This is a formula combining natural botanical extracts and polyphenols to support healthy cell proliferation. Alpha CRS+® contains boswellic acids; silymarin; curcumin; ginkgo; bromelain enzyme; carotenoids; and polyphenols including resveratrol, ellagic acid, baicalin and proanthocyanidins from grape seeds. Alpha CRS+® is formulated to be used daily with xEO Mega and Microplex VMz® as a comprehensive dietary supplement foundation. From this bottle, participants will take two capsules in the morning with breakfast and two capsules in the evening with dinner.

xEO Mega ESSENTIAL OIL OMEGA COMPLEX
dōTERRA's xEO Mega Essential Oil Omega Complex is a formula of Certified Pure Therapeutic Grade® (CPTG) essential

oils and a proprietary blend of marine and land-sourced omega fatty acids. A single daily dose of xEO Mega provides 1000 milligrams of marine lipids with 340 mg EPA, 240 mg DHA, and a blend of plant-sourced essential fatty acids. xEO Mega also includes 800 IU of natural vitamin D, 60 IU of natural vitamin E, and 1 mg of pure astaxanthin, an antioxidant carotenoid harvested from microalgae. The bioavailability of the xEO Mega formula is enhanced through a nanosomal lipid assimilation system and is encapsulated in SLS-free vegetable capsules. From this bottle, participants will take two capsules in the morning with breakfast, and two capsules in the evening with dinner.

Microplex VMz® MICRONUTRIENT COMPLEX

dōTERRA's Microplex VMz® Food Nutrient Complex is an all-natural, whole-food formula of bioavailable vitamins and minerals that are deficient in our modern diets. The formula includes a balanced blend of essential antioxidant vitamins A, C, and E, and an energy complex of B vitamins presented in a patented glycoprotein matrix. It also contains food-derived minerals of calcium, magnesium, and zinc and 72 organic trace minerals for bone and metabolic health. Microplex VMz® contains dōTERRA's Tummy Tamer™ botanical blend of peppermint, ginger, and caraway to calm the stomach for those who may have experienced stomach upset with other vitamin and mineral products (not sold by dōTERRA). Microplex VMz® is encapsulated using sodium lauryl sulfate-free vegetable capsules, does not contain wheat or dairy products, and does not include any animal products or synthetic ingredients. From this bottle, participants will take two capsules in the morning with breakfast, and two capsules in the evening with dinner.

Design: This was a single group study. Each week, one measure of psychological distress was taken such that each measure was used four times during the study. All measures were collected at the start and the end of the study. Each week during the remainder of the study a new measure was taken, allowing for each measure to be taken twice over a two-month period between the initial evaluation and the final evaluation (where all measures were collected at once).

Standard Measures of Depression and Anxiety: All measures used were self-report questionnaires that deal with life events, frustrations, perceptions of stress, and emotional states. These measures do not deal with traits of emotionality (dispositions), coping skills, social support, or health cognitions. Four standard measures of depression and anxiety were selected for this study: 1) Hospital Anxiety and Depression Scale (HADS), 2) General Health Questionnaire (GHQ-12), 3) Center for Epidemiological Studies Depression Scale (CES-D), and 4) Perceived Stress Scale (PSS).

Results

Of 21 initial participants, one, a woman, withdrew from the study claiming bloating from taking the supplements. Thus, there were 14 women and 6 men over the age of 18 with an average age of 39 to 45. While there were 20 in the study who were asked to complete the measures weekly via online survey, not all 20 followed through and answered each week's survey. Because the data was collected anonymously and the study was voluntary, it was difficult to get all participants to follow through each week (weekly reminders were e-mailed to participants but individual reminder notes or phone calls could not be made to collect missing data since the data was being collected anonymously). Because of this, the number of participants who completed the measures varies from week to week, thus accounting for N not being 20, but 8 or 10 in Tables 1 to 4.

dōTERRA's Lifelong Vitality supplement pack had an effect over time for HADS (P<0.04), GHQ-12 (P<0.0001), CES-D (P<0.041), and PSS (P<0.07) as indicated in Tables 1 to 4, respectively. Means scores for each of the four measurements for depression and anxiety progressively decreased from an initial assessment before LLV and at weekly intervals thereafter until final assessment at end of the study.

Table 1. HADS Results

Time	Mean	Std. Deviation	N
HADS (initial evaluation)	15.50[a]	3.472	10
HADS (week 1 evaluation)	11.20[ab]	4.733	10
HADS (week 5 evaluation)	10.30[b]	4.448	10
HADS (final evaluation)	7.80[c]	4.367	10

[bc]Means with different superscript are statistically different (P<0.05).

Table 2. GHQ Results

Time	Mean	Std. Deviation	N
GHQ (initial evaluation)	25.00a	5.268	9
GHQ-12 (week 2 evaluation)	12.78b	7.049	9
GHQ12 (week 6 evaluation)	12.22b	7.839	9
GHQ12 (final evaluation)	9.11b	4.343	9

[ab]Means with different superscript are statistically different (P<0.05).

Table 3. CES-D Results

Time	Mean	Std. Deviation	N
CES-D (initial evaluation)	34.38a	11.807	8
CES-D (week 3 evaluation)	23.62a	11.070	8
CES-D (week 7 evaluation)	18.88a	12.966	8
CES-D (final evaluation)	13.87a	12.403	8

[a]Means with different superscript are statistically different (P<0.05).

Table 4. PSS Results

Time	Mean	Std. Deviation	N
PSS (initial evaluation)	34.11a	5.776	9
PSS (week 4 evaluation)	29.67ab	9.260	9
PSS (week 8 evaluation)	27.56b	7.828	9
PSS (final evaluation)	25.67ab	10.607	9

abMeans with different superscript are statistically different (P<0.05).

There were positive and significant correlations (range, r=0.480 to 0.704, P<0.019 to 0.0001) among the 4 measures as indicated in Table 5.

Table 5. Depression Measures of Correlation Matrix (N=19)

	Hadsinit	GHQinit	CESinit	PSSinit
HADSinit Pearson Correlation Sig. (1-tailed)				
GHQinit Pearson Correlation Sig. (1-tailed)	.704** .000			
CESinit Pearson Correlation Sig. (1-tailed)	.622** .002	.590** .004		
PSSinit Pearson Correlation Sig. (1-tailed)	.534** .009	.480* .019	.525* .010	

Estimated Marginal Means of MEASURE_1

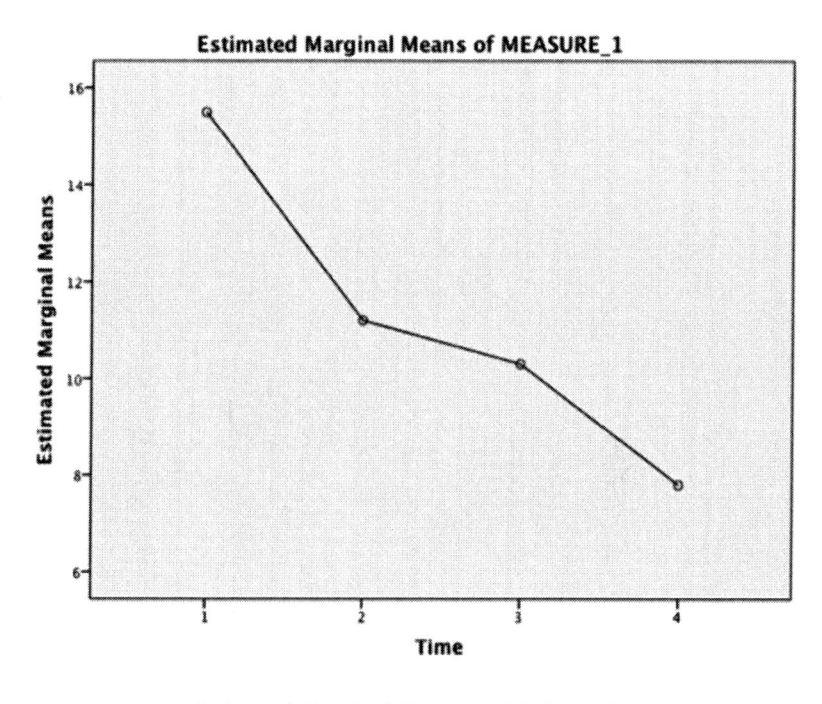

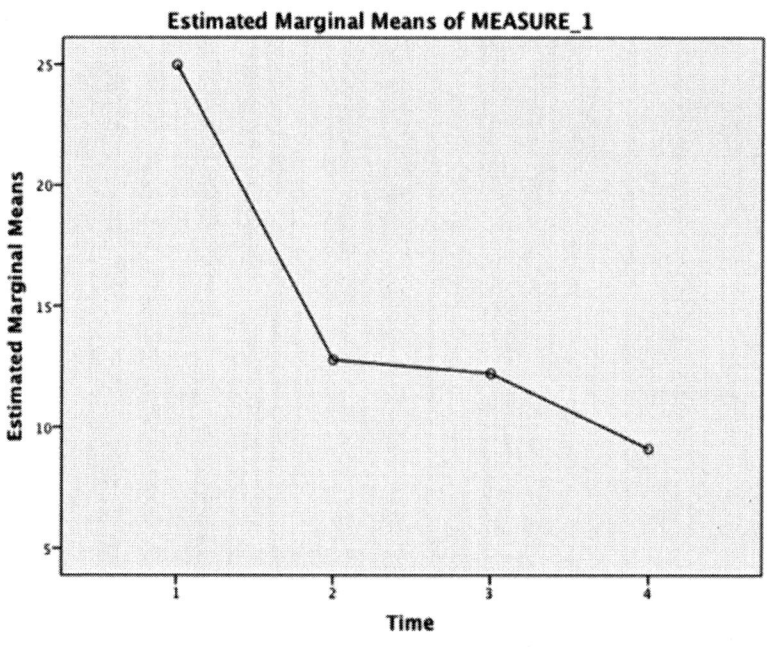

Estimated Marginal Means of MEASURE_1

Estimated Marginal Means of MEASURE_1

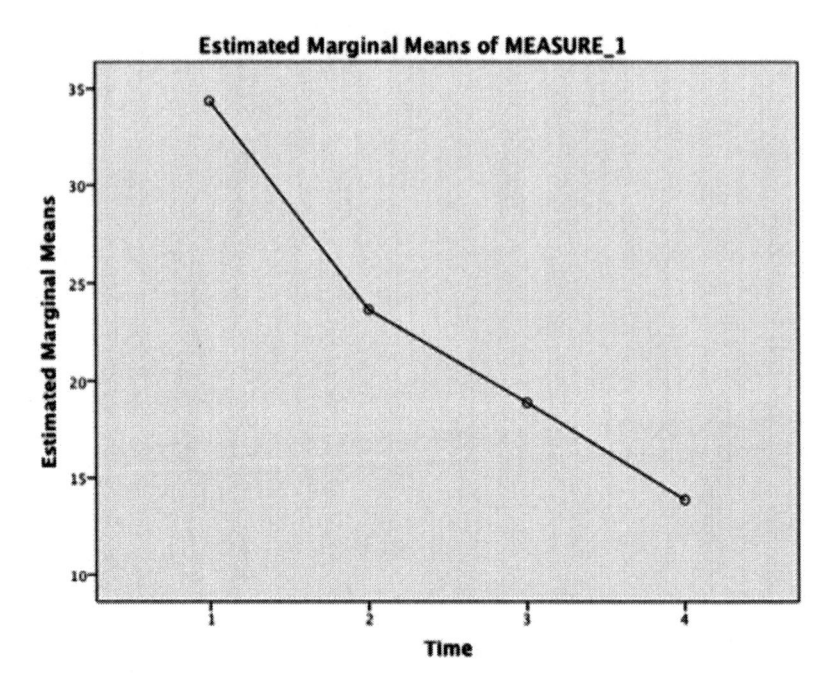

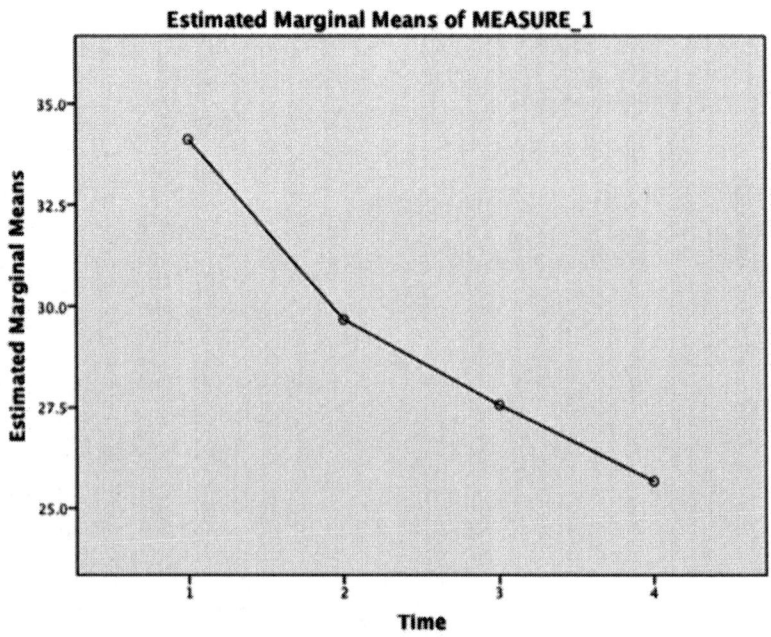

Estimated Marginal Means of MEASURE_1

Discussion

In a December 2012 review study in the *Journal of Medicine and Life* titled "Nutrition and depression at the forefront of progress", authors Maria Ladea and Teodora Popa of the Clinical Hospital of Psychiatry in Bucharest, Romania, wrote that depression is undeniably linked to nutrition, as suggested by the mounting evidence of research in neuropsychiatry. An adequate intake of good calories, healthy proteins, omega-3 fatty acids, and all essential minerals is of utmost importance in maintaining good mental health. In addition, the link between fast food and depression has recently been confirmed. The mounting scientific evidence clearly indicates that the global epidemic of depression and anxiety, which has been growing exponentially over the past three decades, may be linked to diet or nutritional deficiencies.

Why would nutrition affect depression? Neurotransmission plays a role in mood. Neurotransmission is a process that is dependent on having sufficient nutrition for the body to manufacture neurotransmitters such as serotonin, dopamine, norepinephrine, acetylcholine, and glutamate. This study looked at different nutritional contributors to healthy brain function. A partial list of nutrients required for synthesis of neurotransmitters includes amino acids (tryptophan, tyrosine, glutamine), minerals (zinc, copper, iron, magnesium), and B-vitamins (B6, B12, folic acid).

Not having proper nutrition is directly related to depression (Villegas et al, 2011). According to a recent study headed by scientists from the University of Las Palmas de Gran Canaria and the University of Granada, eating commercial baked goods (cakes, croissants, doughnuts, etc.) and fast food (hamburgers, hotdogs and pizza) is linked to depression. The results of a study headed by Almudena Sanchez-Villegas was published in the *Public Health Nutrition* journal and reveal that consumers of fast food (compared to those who eat little or no fast food) are 51 percent more likely to develop depression. Furthermore, a dose-response relationship was recognized suggesting that the more fast food one consumes, the more at risk they are of depression.

Eating healthy, nutrient-packed foods is vital to neurotransmitter function. In order for the body to make neurotransmitters, it must 'gather' the necessary ingredients and have the correct cofactors. This allows for the action of the neurotransmitter to be efficient and effective. Let's take zinc as an example. Zinc is present in particularly large concentrations in the mammalian brain. Brain zinc is located in pre-synaptic terminals. Adequate levels of zinc are necessary for action of synaptic vesicles in some gluatamatergic and serotonergic neurons. It is released with neural activity, probably as a modulator of synaptic transition.

In teens experiencing a growth spurt, zinc is taken to the bones for growth, thereby depleting the nutrient's levels in the brain; this reduces serotonin function at the receptor. Clinically, this will be seen as irritability, depression, acne, and zinc spots (white spots) on nails (Maes, et al, 1994). According to Maes, "lower serum zinc in major depression is a sensitive marker of treatment resistance and of the immune/inflammatory response in that illness." Additionally, in animal models of zinc deficiency there is impairment of whole body accumulation of Omega 3 polyunsaturated fatty acids. On the other hand, excess levels of zinc are associated with neuronal loss (Coppen, 2000), and zinc levels fluctuate inversely with copper levels. Because of this, proper, balanced levels of zinc are important.

Balance is a key in the nutritional path. Omega-3 fatty acids are known to support proper brain function. Dr. Rossella

Liperoti and colleagues at the Catholic University of the Sacred Heart in Rome, Italy, explain that the Omega-3 fatty acids eicosapentaeoic acid (EPA) and docosahexaenoic acid (DHA) are the most common polyunsaturated fatty acids in the brain. These compounds help regulate cell membranes, dopamine and serotonin levels, communication between brain cells, and brain glucose metabolism. As more research is done, evidence demonstrates the role omega-3 depletion may play in several disorders (Liperoti, 2009).

Omega-3s are also significant for both pregnant mothers and infants. It has been established that mothers, unborn infants, and new-born babies benefit from a sufficient amount of long-chain fats in their diets (Judge et al, 2011), as long-chain polyunsaturated fatty acids are essential for synaptogenesis, membrane function, and myelination. Also, referring back to the role of zinc, zinc deficiency alters autonomic nervous system regulation and also hippocampal and cerebral development (Ref). Also, iron deficiency alters myelination, monoamine neutrotransmitter synthesis, and hippocampal energy metabolism for the growing foetus (Georgieff, 2007). Protein and copper are important dietary components. Copper is essential for dopamine metabolism, brain-energy metabolism, antioxidant activity and iron accretion (Prohaska & Gybina 2005).

Lifelong Vitality as a Choice
This research looked at Lifelong Vitality and it's affects on depression because this product reported to contained efficacious dosages of key nutritional ingredients including: polyphenols (such as baicain, resveratrol, ellagic acid, proanthocyanidins, silymarin, and curcumin), carotenoids (such as lutein, lycopene and silymarin), protease enzymes, boswellia serrate, astaxanthin carotenoid, land and fish based omega 3's (1000 mg pure fish oil with 340 mg EPA/240mg DHA including omegas from flax seed oil, borage seed oil, cranberry seed oil,

and pomegranate seed), bacopoa monnieri, vitamins (vitamin A, B, C, D, and E), minerals (such as zinc, calcium, magnesium, chromium, selenium, and 75 other trace minerals all delivered in a food matrix with a patented enzyme delivery system), and essential oils (such as clove, thyme, frankincense, ginger, chamomile, and peppermint).

Lifelong Vitality includes key nutritional support already mentioned in this study (omegas, B-vitamins, zinc, etc). In addition, research into other key ingredients showed direct treatment correlations to stress, anxiety, depression, and other mental health disorders (Sathyanaravanan, et al, 2013, Krishnakumar, 2009, Nakagawa, 2011, Umezu, 2012, Moussaieff, et al, 2012).

The ingredient astaxanthin has been shown in studies to support healing of dementia patients (Nakagawa et al, 2011). Polyphenols are shown to help boost the production of brain stem cells (neurogenesis) and they reinforce their multiplicity in various types of neuron cells (Valente, 2009). Bacopa monnieri has been shown to improve cognition because it reduces anxiety. Bacopa monnieri intermingles with the dopamine and serotonergic systems of the body and its primary job is to promote neuron communication. It does this by enhancing communication in the nervous system that increases the growth of nerve endings or dendrites in the brain. Bacopa monnieri is also an antioxidant and it is shown to be a useful nootropic. Both peppermint and chamomile essential oils (aromatic compounds from peppermint and chamomile leaves) have been shown to have CNS stimulant effects (Umezu, 2012) and frankincense essential oil is shown to have antidepressant properties (Moussaieff, et al, 2012).

Lifelong Vitality incorporates a nanosomal lipid assimilation system (patented by dōTERRA) to ensure greater efficiency and utilization of nutrition. This nanosomal lipid assimilation system helps nutrients pass through the intestinal wall, delivering nutrients through the water layer of the gut. This occurs because the ingredients are encapsulated in micells, a hydrophilic structure used to contain the lipophilic structure. This method provides greater surety that the nutrient is received into the lymphatic channel for rapid assimilation. Since lipids have trouble passing through the intestinal wall, greater absorption of nutrients is a unique quality of this particular product (Hill, 2013).

According to dōTERRA's chief medical officer, Dr. David Hill, Lifelong Vitality is also unique in that it uses essential oils and mixes them with both land and sea based fatty acids offering a minimum of ten times the stability. In this case, Dr. Hill indicates that clove essential oil works as a powerful antioxidant, potentially reducing inflammation by an additional thirty percent. German chamomile works as an anti-inflammatory as well, frankincense supports stabilization, and thyme essential oil preserves, protects, and helps to raise levels of DHEA, also supporting brain function.

Dr. Hill said in an online webinar regarding the Lifelong Vitality pack, "The omega 3's are valuable for brain tissue and they support the myelin sheath, and when they are delivered in their most usable form without converting them to another substance, and when they are added with astaxanthin, a cartonoid, they cross blood-brain barrier and become a powerful antioxidant providing additional cellular protection to brain tissues."

In a previous study conducted on Lifelong Vitality, Dr. Troy Parker (the lead researcher who conducted the study) reported that participants who took this particular supplement pack described having more energy, decreased pain, better mental clarity, improved feelings of balance, and increased happiness

(Parker, 2013). This study, combined with the uniqueness of the product, influenced the decision to use Lifelong Vitality for this particular research.

Depression, Obesity, and Systemic Inflammation
Numerous studies have found evidence connecting depression to obesity. Obesity, of course, is linked to nutrition. A meta-analysis of 17 studies on the link between nutrition and obesity—that included a total of 204, 507 participants—determined that obesity increases the risk for depression, and depression is predictive of developing obesity. The association between depression and obesity for females was significantly higher than that for males (de Wit, 2010). While genetic and environmental factors may also contribute to both obesity and depression, this significant correlation between the two should not be ignored.

As further studies review the correlation between obesity and depression, it will be important not to overlook the role of systemic inflammation as a cause for both diseases. To understand how systemic inflammation is caused, some scientists have focused research on cytokines, an expansive group of pleiotropic and redundant polypeptides that play important roles in the function and pathology of the central nervous system. Cytokines are thought to be involved in various central nervous system functions that are dysregulated in major depression. These include sleep, food intake, cognition, behavior, temperature, and neuroendocrine regulation. Likewise, cytokines have been shown to play a role in insulin resistance and increased risk for cardiovascular disease. They also have been proven to cause inflammation within the brain when they are allowed to pass the gut-brain barrier. Researchers at the Clinical Neuroendocrinology Branch of the National Institutes of Health in Bethesda, Maryland have published work linking inflammatory cytokines (especially the IL-1 family) to major depression (Licinio, 1999).

Among other problems linked to systemic inflammation, and possibly depression, are an increase in insulin and leptin hormones, based on a 2003 study concluding that insulin resistance is, at least in part, a chronic inflammatory disease (Xu, 2003). Insulin resistance leads to sympathetic nervous system over-arousal, which in turn can lead to increased cortisol levels and can cause the body to lose magnesium (Takase, 2004). Decreased magnesium can lead to migraines and poor sleep, which are both thought to contribute to episodes of major depression. Where such is the case, the depressed mind may not be affected by serotonin production (which traditional antidepressants work to regulate) but by magnesium deficiencies--again, another link between nutrition and depression.

Lifelong Vitality contains carotenoids (such as Lutein, Lycopene, Silymarin, and Curcumin) which are powerful, free-radical scavengers (reported to be ten times more powerful than vitamin E) and these carotenoids are known to increase glutathione levels in liver, increase superoxide dismutase enzyme, stimulate growth of new liver cells, and mediate inflammatory markers (Hill, 2013). Further research into these vital nutritive elements would be necessary to define a more direct correlation to inflammation, obesity, and mood.

Food intolerances are another likely cause of systemic inflammation. Intolerance to dairy products, legumes, and grains has been shown most often to lead to systemic inflammation. This is typically due to a large population of modern human beings who lack the enzymes capable of breaking down the proline proteins in grains, especially gluten and gliadin. The saponins in legumes and lactose and casein in dairy are also problematic for many people. When undigested particles of poline, gluten, gliadin, saponins, lactose, or casein cross the intestine into the bloodstream, the body treats them like foreign invaders and sends an immune response. That immune response includes inflammatory cytokines, suggesting again that research should look into how these cytokines affect depression and what we should or shouldn't eat to prevent their release.

Another factor to consider is that when cellular mitochondria receive proper nutrition, often the result is a change of interest in diet. It has been reported that proper nutrition that supports the mitochondria results in less interest in foods that are unhealthy (unhealthy carbohydrates and/or foods high in sugar). Lifelong Vitality (and other quality nutritional supplementation) generally support feeding mitochondria and in the process, food interests and choices may be altered or improved by those who take supplements. It's possible that those who take Lifelong Vitality naturally begin to change their interest in certain unhealthy foods and begin making selections that provide better overall nutritional support simply because the body is being properly fed. As a result, the health of other systems of the body may improve (i.e., organ function, cellular repair, healthy weight loss, and inflammatory response) all of which may improve immune function and support overall mood and general well being.

As we look at nutrition for health and well being there are recent research reports that indicate that some commercial agriculture techniques may be leaving the soil where food is grown deficient in important minerals, causing the food that's bought and sold in grocery stores to be mineral deficient (Davis, 2004). A study conducted by Dr. Donald Davis from the University of Texas (USA) Department of Chemistry and Biochemistry found reliable declines over the last fifty years in the amount of protein, calcium, phosphorus, iron, riboflavin (vitamin B2) and vitamin C found in foods. This research suggests that declining nutritional content is caused by a host of agricultural practices created to improve some traits (like size, growth rate, pest management) rather than increase nutritional value. Davis said the following about his study results: "Perhaps more worrisome would be declines in nutrients we could not study because they were not reported in 1950—magnesium, zinc, vitamin B-6, vitamin E and dietary fiber, not to mention phytochemicals." While additional studies in which old and new crop varieties should be looked at side-by-side and measured by modern methods, his research details key nutrients possibly missing in today's foods that are necessary to support healthy mind and mood.

There are other factors that are reported today to affect the quality of food found at local grocery stores. Today, foods are shipped long distances and are stored for long periods of time, both of which may cause depletion of vitamins and minerals, including B-vitamins, needed for brain function and known to support the central nervous system. Some food processing techniques used today deplete nutrients from fruits and vegetables. For example, there are genetically grown crops now that are meant to improve visual appeal and increase harvests, but nutritional value is not necessarily increased in these practices. Also, increased levels of environmental pollution and toxins often cause the body to use more nutrients than normal (such as antioxidants) to detoxify and eliminate harmful substances. All of these factors contribute to why even those who eat a healthy diet may find support from additional targeted nutrition.

The bottom line in the research cited here as well as the results from this study of dōTERRA's Lifelong Vitality pack, is that nutrition and depression have a connection. While depression is complex and not always caused by only one factor, supporting the body by providing adequate nutrition is a positive step in the right direction; and in some cases deficiencies of certain vitamins, minerals, amino acids do directly relate to emotional wellbeing. The impact of diet on depression may have been underestimated or unknown until recently. Nutrition for mental health is one of the important factors that need further consideration and research to adequately address and explain the complexities surrounding nutrition and mental health.

Conclusion

The results of this study submit the possibility that there is a relationship between nutrition (Lifelong Vitality), depression, and anxiety. These results are consistent with other preliminary research on nutrition and depression, including a previously conducted study on Lifelong Vitality (Parker, 2013).

While there are many factors that can contribute to depression (i.e., psychological issues, trauma, family background, life changes, and so forth), there is significant research indicating that here are a number of nutritional factors that can contribute toward depressive symptoms.

We know that depression is not caused by just one factor and research tells us that eating well and supplementing may be a positive step in the right direction. According to NHS's website, we learn that it's possible that deficiencies of certain vitamins, minerals, amino and fatty acids relate to our emotional wellbeing (NHS, 2014). Today, many other medical websites (along with NHS) instruct those with mild depression to look to what they eat to assist symptoms of depression.

"Diet is one of the important factors for our mental health," said Andrew McCulloch, the chief executive at the Mental Health Foundation (Williams, 2014). McCullough, like others, has said that the influence of diet on depression has been undervalued. In the next decade or so, it's anticipated that more research of this kind will yield additional answers for those suffering with mental health disorders. For now, eating a well-balanced, assorted healthy diet that may include a full range of micronutrients, and adding supplementation to a healthy diet may provide beneficial results for more than just mood.

While it's not possible to state for certain that a positive relationship exists between Lifelong Vitality and depression without further research, this preliminary research raises interest in a growing area of research and heightens awareness in the possibility that Lifelong Vitality may support individuals suffering from depression and anxiety.

References

Blom, HJ, & Smulders, Y., (2011). *Overview of homocysteine and folate metabolism.* Journal of Inherited Metabolic Disease. 34(1): 75–81.

California Institute of Technology, (2013). *Probiotic therapy alleviates autism-like behaviors in mice.* ScienceDaily. Retrieved August 20, 2014 from www.sciencedaily.com/releases/2013/12/131205141900.htm.

Cohen, S., Karmarck, T., & Mermelstein, R., (1983). *A global measure of perceived stress.* Journal of Health and Social Behaviour, 24, 385-396.

Coppen A, and Bailey J, (2000). *Enhancement of the antidepressant action of fluoxetine by folic acid: a randomised, placebo controlled trial.* J Affect Disord 2000; 60:121–130.

Davis, D., (2009). *Declining Fruit and Vegetable Nutrient Composition: What Is the Evidence?* HortScience, vol. 44 no. 1:15-19.

deWit, et al., (2010). *Depression and obesity: A meta-analysis of community-based studies.* Psychiatry Research. 178(2); 230–35.

dōTERRA corporation, (2014). dōTERRA published corporate product pages, http://www.dōTERRAtools.com/lifelong-vitality-products/

Fobbester, D. et al., (2004). Optimum Nutrition UK survey. Available from www.ion.ac.uk

Gilbody, et al. (2007). *Methylenetetrahydrofolate Reductase (MTHFR) Genetic Polymorphisms (C677T variant) and Psychiatric Disorders: A HuGE Review.* Am J Epidemiol 2007;165:1–13.

Goldberg, D.P, (1978). Reproduced by NFER-NELSON. This measure is part of *Measures in Health Psychology: A Users Portfolio,* written and compiled by Professor Marie Johnston, Dr. Stephen Wright, and Professor John Winman.

Goldberg, D.P., et al (1997). *The validity of two versions of the GHQ in the WHO study of mental illness in general health care.* Psychological Medicine, 27: 191-197.

Hill, D. (2013). *dōTERRA - Essential Fatty Acids, Vitamins & Minerals With Dr. Hill,* lecture recorded and placed on youtube: http://www.youtube.com/watch?v=t-Iv7iCq0q0

Holford, P. (2003). *Depression: the nutrition connection.* Primary Care Mental Health. 1: 9–16.

Journal of Trauma, vol. 68, no 5 (2010): pp. 1059–64.

Kang, H. J., et al. (2012). *Decreased expression of synapse-related genes and loss of synapses in major depressive disorder.* Nature Medicine. 18 1413–17.

Kessler, R., et al. (2005). *Prevalence, severity, and comorbidity of twelve-month DSM-IV disorders in the National Comorbidity Survey Replication (NCS-R).* Archives of General Psychiatry, 2005 Jun; 62(6):617-27.

Krishnakumar, et al. (2009). *Upregulation of 5-HT2C receptors in hippocampus of pilocarpine-induced epileptic rats: antagonism by Bacopa monnieri,* Epilepsy Behav. 2009 Oct;16(2):225-30. doi: 10.1016/j.yebeh.2009.07.031. Epub 2009 Aug 22.

Lespérance, F., et al. (2010). *The Efficacy of Omega-3 Supplementation for Major Depression: A Randomized Controlled Trial.* Journal of Clinical Psychiatry; DOI: 10.4088/JCP.10m05966blu

Licinio, J., and Wong, M-L., (1999). *The role of inflammatory mediators in the biology of major depression: central nervous system cytokines modulate the biological substrate of depressive symptoms, regulate stress-responsive systems, and contribute to neurotoxicity and neuroprotection.* Molecular Psychiatry. 4; 317–27.

Liperoti, R., et al. (2009). *Omega-3 polyunsaturated fatty acids and depression: a review of the evidence.* Current Pharmaceutical Design, Vol. 15, December 2009, pp. 4165-72.

Lyte, M., (2011). *Probiotics function mechanistically as delivery vehicles for neuroactive compounds: Microbial endocrinology in the design and use of probiotics.* BioEssays. 33(8):574–81.

Maes, M., et al. (1994). *Hypozincemia in depression.* J Affective Disorders; 31(2):13.

Maes, M. (1997). *Lower serum zinc in major depression is a sensitive marker of treatment resistance and of the immune/inflammatory response in that illness.* Biol Psychiatry: 42(5):349-358

Maes, M, et.al. (1999). *Lower serum zinc in major depression in relation to changes in serum acute phase proteins.* J. Affect Disord 1999:56(2-3):189-194

Mayer, E. (2011). *Gut feelings: the emerging biology of gut-brain communication.* www.nature.com/reviews/neuro. Retrieved August 17, 2014.

Miller, et al. (2010). *Clinical and biochemical effects of catecholamine depletion on antidepressant-induced remission of depression.* Arch Gen Psychiatry. Vol.53(2):117-128.

Moussaieff, et al. (2012). *Incensole acetate reduces depressive-like behavior and modulates hippocampal BDNF and CRF expression of submissive animals.* J Psychopharmacol. 2012 Dec;26(12):1584-93. doi: 10.1177/0269881112458729. Epub 2012 Sep 26.

Nakagawa et al. (2011). *Antioxidant effect of astaxanthin on phospholipid peroxidation in human erythrocytes.* Br J Nutr. 2011 Jun;105(11):1563-71. doi: 10.1017/S0007114510005398. Epub 2011 Jan 31.

National Health Services (NHS) (2014). *Healthy Eating and Depression.* Published online, last review, June, 2014, http://www.nhs.uk/Conditions/stress-anxiety-depression/Pages/healthy-diet-depression.aspx

Nierenberg et al. (2011). *The current crisis of confidence in antidepressants.* J Clin Psychiatry 2011; 72:27–33.

Parker, T. (2013). *Quantitative and qualitative evaluation of a multi-component supplement: a preliminary human clinical trial on dōTERRA's Lifelong Vitality Pack.* Published online at: http://www.agoodchange.com/wp-content/uploads/2013/10/LifelongVitalityPackStudy.pdf

Radloff, L.S. (1977). *The CES-D scale: A self-report depression scale for research in the general population.* Applied Psychological Measurement 1: 385-401.

Ruusunen, A. (2013). *Diet and depression.* Publications of the University of Eastern Finland. Dissertations in Health Sciences, no 185.

Sánchez-Villegas, A., et al (2011). *Fast-food and commercial baked goods consumption and the risk of depression.* Public Health Nutrition, 2011; 15 (03): 424 DOI: 10.1017/S1368980011001856

Sathyanarayanan, et al, (2013). *Brahmi for the better? New findings challenging cognition and anti-anxiety effects of Brahmi (Bacopa monniera) in healthy adults.* Psychopharmacology (Berl), 227(2):99-306. doi: 10.1007/s00213-013-2978-z. Epub 2013 Jan 26.

Self, A., Thomas, J and Randall, C. (2012). *Measuring National Well-being: Life in the UK.* 2012 Office for National Statistics, 20 November 2012, Office for National Statistics.

Spillmann, et.al. (2001). *Tryptophan depletion in SSRI recovered depressed outpatients.* Psychopharmacology (Berl), May;155 (2):123-127.

Stanway, A. (1981). *Overcoming Depression.* Hamlyn Publishing Group, Ltd.

Takase, B. (2004). *Effect of chronic stress and sleep deprivation on both flow-mediated dilation in the brachial artery and the intracellular magnesium level in humans.* Clinical Cardiology. Retrieved on March 15, 2012.

Thase, M.E. (2003). *Effectiveness of antidepressants: comparative remission rates.* J. Clin Psychiatry. 64:3–7.

Tillisch, K., et al, (2013). *Consumption of fermented milk product with probiotic modulates brain activity.* Gastroenterology. June; 1444(7):1394–401.

Umezu T. (2012). *Evaluation of the Effects of Plant-derived Essential Oils on Central Nervous System Function Using Discrete Shuttle-type Conditioned Avoidance Response in Mice.* Phytother Res. Phytother Res. 2012;26(6):884-891.

Valente, et al. (2009). *A Diet Enriched in Polyphenols and Polyunsaturated Fatty Acids, LMN Diet, Induces Neurogenesis in the Subventricular Zone and Hippocampus of Adult Mouse Brain.* Journal of Alzheimer's Disease, 2009; 18 (4) DOI: 10.3233/JAD-2009-118

Walsh BT, et al, (2002). *Placebo response in studies of major depression: variable, substantial, and growing.* JAMA. 2002 Apr 10;287(14):1840-7

Williams, H. (2014). *How to beat depression with the right diet,* Independent.co.uk, http://www.independent.co.uk/life-style/health-and-families/features/how-to-beat-depression-with-the-right-diet-1817675.html

Xu, H. (2003). *Chronic inflammation in fat plays a crucial role in the development of obesity-related insulin resistance.* The Journal of Clinical Investigation. Retrieved on March 15, 2012.

Young, S. (2007). *Folate and depression—a neglected problem.* J Psychiatry Neurosci 32(2):80–2

Young, S. (2007). *How to increase serotonin in the human brain without drugs.* J Psychiatry Neurosci 32(6):394–99

Zigmund and Snaith, (1983). From "The Hospital Anxiety and Depression Scale," Acta Psychiatrica Scandinavica 67, 361-70. Published by the NFER-NELSON Publishing Company Ltd, Darville House, 2 Oxford Road East, Windsor, Berkshire SL4 1DF, UK

Zorc, et al, (1991). *Expenditures for psychotropic medications in the United States in 1985.* Am J Psychiatry. May;148(5):644-7.